If ever I was conceited, that was driven out of me one evening long ago when a widow came and begged me to help her daughter who, she said, was dying. I went with her and found on the floor, kicking and screaming, a hysterical girl. The minute she saw me she said to her mother, "I won't have that doctor — you send for my doctor!" The mother said, "Shut up — at a time like this you take any damn thing you can get!"

ALVAREZ ON ALVAREZ

Walter Clement Alvarez, M.D.

Strawberry Hill Press

ALVAREZ ON ALVAREZ

Strawberry Hill Press
616 44th Avenue
San Francisco, California 94121

Distributed by Stackpole Books
Cameron & Kelker Sts.
Harrisburg, Pennsylvania 17105

Book edited by Scott Lowe

First Printing, December, 1977

Manufactured in the United States of America

Library of Congress Cataloging in Publication Data

Alvarez, Walter Clement, 1884-
Alvarez on Alvarez.

Bibliography: p.
1. Alvarez, Walter Clement, 1884-
2. Physicians—United States—Biography. I. Title.
R154.A545A28 610'.92'4 (B) 76-47216
ISBN 0-89407-005-3 (Strawberry)

A PARTIAL LIST OF BOOKS BY
Walter C. Alvarez, M.D.

DANGER SIGNALS Chicago: Follett, 1953
HELP YOUR DOCTOR HELP YOU Millbrae, CA.: Celestial Arts, 1976
INCURABLE PHYSICIAN Englewood Cliffs, N.J.: Prentice-Hall, 1963
AN INTRODUCTION TO GASTROENTEROLOGY New York: Paul Hoeber, 1940
LITTLE STROKES Philadelphia: J.B. Lippincott Company, 1966
LIVE AT PEACE WITH YOUR NERVES Englewood Cliffs, N.J.: Prentice-Hall, 1958
THE MECHANICS OF THE DIGESTIVE TRACE New York: Paul Hoeber, 1922; Second Ed., 1928
MINDS THAT CAME BACK Philadelphia: J.B. Lippincott Company, 1961
NERVES IN COLLISION New York: Pyramid Publications, 1972
NERVOUS INDIGESTION New York: Paul Hoeber, 1930
NERVOUSNESS, INDIGESTION AND PAIN New York: Paul Hoeber, 1943
THE NEUROSES Philadelphia: W.B. Saunders Company, 1951
PRACTICAL LEADS TO PUZZLING DIAGNOSES Philadelphia: J.B. Lippincott Company, 1958
WALTER C. ALVAREZ ON LIFE & HEALTH Chatsworth, CA.: Major Books, 1975

TABLE OF CONTENTS

INTRODUCTION

I. MY FAMILY BACKGROUND

II. 1888-1895

III. 1895-1901

IV. 1901-1905

V. 1905-1906

VI. 1907-1909

VII. 1910-1913

VIII. 1913-1926

IX. 1926-1950

X. THE DOCTORS MAYO

XI. 1950-1975

XII. THE FAITH OF A PHYSICIAN

XIII. THOUGHTS ON THE THEORY OF EVOLUTION

POST SCRIPT

INTRODUCTION

In 1963 my autobiography, *Incurable Physician,* was published. At the time I was a young 79-years, had recently "retired" from the Mayo Clinic, and was practicing medicine in Chicago. Today, 14 years later, I believe it is time to "up-date" the story of my life — not for myself so much as for the general public with which I still have so much close contact and for the young physicians of today who appear to view medicine as I did: a way to help people. For me, as for them, medicine must be a kindly art.

My friend, Dr. Gregg of the Rockefeller Institute, told me that his talks with hundreds of students of medicine and science, in America, in Europe, and in Asia, showed him how hungry they were to know how to succeed intellectually, socially, emotionally and spiritually.

How to climb the ladder of success? When and how to learn the need for absolute honesty in observation and thinking? When does one get the courage to criticize unwise medical practices — the strength to stand up firmly in the face of opposition and, perhaps, bitter and unfair criticism? When and why decide to remain at work when you know that your opponents will ignore — never mention — the work you did?

"In your book, Walter, you must tell your readers that you ran into opposition — but you kept going. Then people everywhere will feel less alone, because they will know that theirs is a common experience."

I hope that my life story will strengthen the determination of younger physicians and surgeons to stick with their resolve to never practice medicine just as a means to make money, but always as a means of greatly helping thousands of suffering fellow men and women.

I have always found it helpful to call on and make friends with others who have done fine work in the field. For example, when Banting and Best reported their discovery of insulin, I went to Toronto — to their laboratory — where I had some grand chats with them both. And when Dr. Fleming, the discoverer of penicillin, came to America for a long visit, I had several happy dinners with him. I found that these people were happy to share their views with me, as I have always tried to share my views with the men and women of our profession who contacted me. One of the things I marvelled at scores of times was the willingness of great physicians to entrust me with secrets which, had I "spilled" them, might have caused much trouble.

There have been many changes in the practice of medicine since I was a boy of ten, 83 years ago. I recall my father making his calls on horseback or in a little buggy. I saw his first operation, about 1888, performed on our kitchen table; with the local minister giving the anesthetic — well-watched by Dad — and with my mother acting as nurse. Later, in Honolulu, I saw operations performed by surgeons dressed in Prince Albert coats, without masks or gloves. In my own Honolulu days, from around 1896 to 1901, so far as I know, the several doctors in that city never had a meeting together. Even in San Francisco in the early days of this century, none of the professors in the four medical schools there at the time would visit another school.

Roentgen reported his discovery of X-rays in December, 1895. But, in 1905 when I went to work in a big City and County Hospital, I found only a small, almost useless X-ray apparatus in a small room near the wards of Cooper College.

I marvel that my father was able to practice medicine in 1888 without any of the splendid drugs we have today. He told me that when he was a boy, in about 1860, he got a fever and heard his own father send a messenger for a doctor. My father jumped out a window and hid in the nearby woods, because he knew that the only things the doctor would do would be to bleed him and purge him — and he didn't want those futile treatments. In fact, he recovered nicely without them!

One reason I can write about the many changes in medicine is that since 1904 I have kept a diary. Before writing *Incurable Physician* I consulted 62 of those diaries, and I spent months dictating notes about the more interesting comments I had recorded.

I hope that in all of this, and with the frequent use of "I," I do not sound too conceited. If ever I was conceited, it was driven out of me one evening long ago when a neighbor came to me, begging me to go to her house to help her daughter "who was dying." I went with her to find, on the floor, kicking and screaming, a hysterical girl. The moment she saw me she screamed at her mother, "I won't have that doctor — you send for *my* doctor." With which the mother retorted: "Shut up. At a time like this you take any damn thing you can get!"

The Broadmoor
San Francisco
September, 1977

CHAPTER I

My Family Background

I am a great believer in the outstanding value to a man or woman of a good ancestry. Fine, able, gifted, sane and industrious ancestors are a great heritage. And so I will tell here of what little I know about my ancestry, and give a brief outline of how my family now stands.

I wish I knew more about my grandparents, but I never saw them, and both my parents were reticent about their forebears and their early days. My father, Luis Fernandez Alvarez, was born on April 1, 1853 in the province of Asturias, Spain. Asturias borders on the Bay of Biscay. Perhaps because that part of Spain was conquered by the Goths around 400 A.D., my father was blue-eyed and very industrious. When he was a boy he very much wanted to receive good schooling, particularly in the area of scientific knowledge. Such training was denied him because the only school near where he lived was very inadequate; little was taught there other than religion.

What little I know of my grandfather consists in the knowledge that he must have been very able because he was chosen to be manager of the palace and the business of Don Francisco de Paula, a "younger son" of the Spanish king, Carlos IV. The Prince respected my grandfather so much that he promised to educate my father and his brothers in the Royal School of Madrid. My uncle Anthony, who was blond and handsome, was educated there. But when it came my father's turn, the local clergy, apparently reluctant to educate such a bright and ambitious lad, managed to block his entrance into the Royal School. Some time before this, my grandfather had died after an unfortunate accident — as a "joke," he was pushed from a balcony. My father was so frantic for a good education that after six months his older brother Constantino took him to Havana, Cuba. That occurred in 1866, when he was only thirteen years old. And so he left Spain, leaving behind his step-mother and step-sister. Because my father and his brother Anthony had no desire to remain in Spain and run the ranch that had been owned by their now deceased father, they gave it to Constantino.

My father found a good way to earn a living in Cuba while continuing his education: each day he read educational books to a big room full of cigar makers, who would then pay him for saving them from boredom as they worked! After some years he left Havana and went to New York where he got a remunerative job and a place to study.

My mother's grandparents had settled many years before in St. Paul, Minnesota. My mother's grandfather, from all accounts a very intelligent man, had been a wealthy vineyardist in Germany before sailing for America. My grandmother was a devoted Catholic, and so loved her priest — Father Clement — that she named my mother Clementina (and I, in turn, was dubbed Walter Clement).

It happened that my father left New York for St. Paul, and it was there that he first saw my mother. Partly because she looked so Spanish, and partly because of their natural attraction for each other, he soon got her to marry him.

In about 1880, they moved to Los Angeles, Califonia. Three years later Dad owned a block of what is now downtown Los Angeles. The river went dry and, unable to foresee the massive aqueducts which now bring rivers of water to the city, he believed there could never be a growing city there. So he sold his property and moved again, this time to San Francisco, where in 1885 he began his medical education in Cooper College.

He graduated in 1887 and opened an office in San Francisco; not knowing many people there, he had little success. When he told one of his old professors about his anxiety over this, the man said, "I can give you the job of doctor aboard a steamer going to Hawaii. It leaves tomorrow!" My father accepted the offer.

I am fortunate in that my father and my mother were the outstading members of their respective families. My mother was attractive, a fine conversationalist, as well as an excellent writer who was always interested in self-improvement. She was a bit nervous, however, and suffered at times from migraine headaches. She inherited the familial passion for music — she had three close relatives who were professional musicians. (I remember her saying one day to my father, "Lu, Lu, I cannot bear any longer being without music; please get me a piano." He did! And by herself, she learned to play it.) As soon as we were in Honolulu she found a good voice teacher, and from that time on, for the rest of her days, she trained her voice and loved to sing. She was alto in a big church.

My parents' first child was a boy who, at age four, died of the awful disease diphtheria. I was born in San Francisco on July 22, 1884. My brother Milton, my two sisters, Florence and Mabel, and my younger brother Harold were all born later.

Milton resided in the Phillipines, where he married a Moro princess and became a buyer of copra, a dried coconut meat from which coconut oil is extracted. The Moros were so pleased with Milton that when their Raja died, they asked if he would be interested in performing the same governmental functions that the Raja did prior to his death. Milton did not think it wise to take such a step at that time and so did not accept their offer. He died at the early age of 35.

Florence was an excellent school teacher, a person who all her life has been motivated to help others. She ceased to teach after she married. My sister Mabel is a splendid artist, and art has kept her busy all her days. Harold, a big, fine-looking man, was at one time Professor of Dental Surgery at the University of California and had a large practice in San Francisco. He is now retired. He and his lovely wife have one son, Richard, an able scientist.

In February, 1907, I married Harriet Smyth, a graduate of U.C.

Berkeley. We have four children, all of whom have been a delight. I am glad to say that I have been happy in the successes of both my children and the offspring of my children.

My eldest child is Gladys, a graduate of the University of California. When she was secretary to that great man, Professor Herbert Evans, he once told me that she had the best mind of any woman he knew. Her first husband, Dr. Raymond C. Archibald, died a few years ago. Their marriage produced a beautiful daughter, Kit. Gladys has since remarried to a fine man, Mr. A. J. Muirhead.

My elder son Luis graduated with a doctorate degree from the University of Chicago. Shortly after graduation, he went to work with the great physicist, Earnest Lawrence at the University of California. There he became a professor of Physics, and took part in the making of the atom bomb. In 1958, he had the great honor of receiving the Nobel Prize for Physics. Luis has been married twice and has four wonderful children. His son Walter has done excellent work in geological research, and has written a book on the subject.

My son Robert also holds a doctorate, and has been the head of three large libraries. He presently publishes *Administrator's Digest,* a journal that goes every month to head librarians and executives around the country. Robert and his wife have three children.

My daughter Bernice, a college graduate, is married to a physician of high repute, Dr. Bradley Brownson. She is a skillful artist and photographer. She and her husband have four children.

CHAPTER II

1888-1895

Early in 1888, when I was three years old, my father moved to Hawaii with my mother, baby Milton and me. Dad was promptly given a position as Government physician, and after a few months in Waianae, we moved to a larger village called Waialua, located twenty-eight miles west of Honolulu.

There we lived in a deserted old Mission church, with the three room parsonage under the same roof as the big hall. There was a nice spring, a well, an outdoor toilet, a farm house, and a servant house. For eight years I slept at night on a couch in the church!

My father became responsible for the health of the natives and foreign workers on a few sugar plantations. Every so often he had to travel, in a buggy, fifty miles along a road running along a narrow shelf between the ocean and the central range of mountains.

We were largely isolated from the world. The only non-Hawaiian and non-Oriental people who occasionally visited us were the English Halsteads, who owned the big sugar plantation a mile or two east of us. There were a few English and American people in the neighborhood, and several hermits who never came near us. Three men who lived alone near the beach in small shacks were "outcasts" who received money from their families in England. One of them told Dad that his father was a knight and he, the hermit, was a graduate of Oxford.

An Englishman who was head of tne native school, located only a few yards from our house, never, so far as I can remember, came to our door. Just north of us was a friendly Hawaiian family, and across the street was a Chinese family, but none of those people ever came into our yard either.

In my boyhood I doubt if any native would work in a cane field, but some worked on ships on the wharves, or on the ranches. They fished, but never sold the fish. If they ever had a fish to spare, they loved to give it to a passing American. They seemed to dread only one sin, and that was selfishness.

On day the handsome local Hawaiian minister came to my father and asked, "Doctor, do you think my wife is beautiful?" And my father said, "Yes, she is very beautiful." The minister said, "That settles it. To show that I am not cursed with selfishness, I must share her sexually with my best friend." As was to be expected, the American bishop fired the man, but many Hawaiians rallied to his support, and got for him a bigger and finer church in Honolulu.

When I was five, my mother quickly taught me to read, and soon I was searching the house hoping to find something to read. Unfortunately for me, my father was never much of a book buyer, and in Waialua we had no newspaper and no journals. The Halsteads were very kind, sometimes bringing me British children's journals. At my urgent request, my father once bought me a book on science and some carpenter's tools.

At age seven, I was given Mother's old catechism and told to memorize it. I read it, and then said, "Mother, the man who wrote that evidently thought he knew all about life in heaven, but he was never there, so he could not have known what goes on. So I don't want to have anything more to do with the booklet." Mother very wisely put it away.

An early sign of the future research scientist in me came one day when I started to take a sliver out of my finger with a pin. My mother immediately said, "Don't do that, Walter, use a needle." I asked, "But why?" And mother said, "Because the pin is brass and the needle is iron." But again I asked, "But what is the difference?" Mother could not explain, and so for years I kept asking elderly men and women and some doctors about the pin and needle. They all agreed that my mother had been right, but could not tell me why.

I learned something when I asked farmers why they nailed an old horseshoe above their barn doors. They said that iron keeps wicked elves from riding the horses all night, and wearing them out! There was also some belief that an iron needle could keep elves from infecting a scratched hand.

My father was a good companion; he made me happy by his constant kindliness, good humor, love of fun, and his love of teaching me things. At an early age I began to learn Spanish from him.

One day as we drove in Dad's little buggy, we passed a Hawaiian man, wearing only a new denim shirt. My father said, "Look, Walter, someone gave that native a new shirt, and he so quickly rushed out to show it to the neighbors that he forgot to put on his pants!"

I loved to go on moonlight nights to a beautiful beach where the waves moved incessantly and the little crabs kept running around. I loved the beautiful double rainbows of Hawaii, and the big clouds on the 4000-foot mountain, Kaala, just east of us. Years later I climbed it to the top.

One fact I now marvel at is that in my mind's eye I can still see many scenes that I saw when I was three years old! How can tiny cells in my brain have retained those pictures?

I can remember how some natives in the schoolyard next door gave a luau, or feast. First they dug a little pit and lined it with stones. They then put wood into the pit and set the wood afire. They then took out the ashes and lined the pit with big "ti" leaves. Next they cut up meat and other foods into fist-sized packages, covered them with ti leaves, and put the packages into the hot pit. They covered it with ti leaves and a gunny sack, and poured in water which, on the hot rocks, made steam — which cooked the food. The guests sat on the ground and ate with their fingers.

Very fortunately for me and the family, my father escaped miraculously from two bad accidents and a pneumonia. Once, in a severe rainstorm, he tried on horseback to cross a flooded river. When his horse stumbled and threw him into the water, all that saved him from drowning was the presence of two native cowboys who threw him a rope and pulled him out. The second accident occurred when a steer

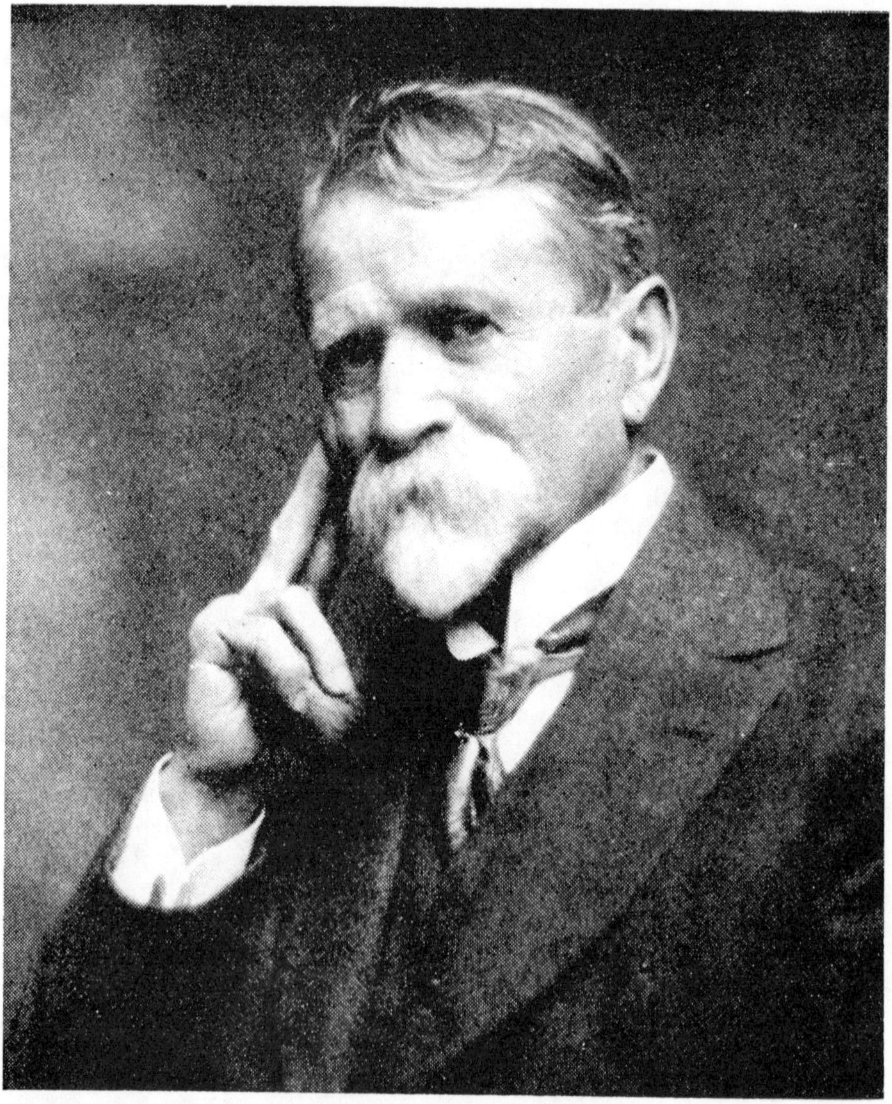

My father, Luis F. Alvarez

on the road tried to gore my father's horse. The horse ran out of control and toppled with Dad over a ten-foot ridge onto the beach. Luckily at that point there was sand, which broke my father's fall, so he was not injured. Our family was saved from disaster when my father came down with severe pneumonia and was given up as "almost dead" by the attending physician. But then, suddenly and miraculously, he recovered. "Where's my breakfast?," he boomed.

One day when I was five or six, bathing with my father in the ocean, I slipped on some seaweed and fell on some sharp coral which cut the skin of my left temple and made it bleed. When my father said he would have to put in some stitches, I cried all the way home. But when Dad started sewing, and I found the pain was bearable, I stopped crying. My father said, "You see, Walter, you have now learned one of the useful lessons in life. Often the anticiption of evil hurts us more than does the evil when it arrives."

One day, when I was nine, I asked my father "How did that black cow get into the yard next door?" And he said, "That is a Japanese photographer with camera and tripod, and a black cloth over his head." Of course, he then realized that my vision was bad, and so he soon drove me around the island and down Nuuanu valley to Honolulu where, fortunately, I got some eye glasses.

Along the road, my father called my attention to plover birds on the beach, and told me that, all by themselves, they had flown to Hawaii from the Aleutian islands near Alaska. I read recently that what Dad said is true, that some of those birds in winter continue to fly down as far as New Zealand. I still wonder how birds could have been given the knowledge that Hawaii exists, where it is, and how to fly there — over some two thousand miles of ocean.

One day, about 1889, my father took me to see an American who had brought to Waialua what he said was the first Edison phonograph. The music was not very loud, nor very clear, but it seemed to me to be miraculous.

It was in Hawaii that I first discovered the tremendous influence of the power of the mind over the body. That discovery still influences me much today. My father saw a number of cases in which a Kahuna, or native witch doctor, "prayed someone to death." As soon as a native heard what the Kahuna was doing to him, he would sit down, stop eating, and in a week or ten days would be dead. My father tried hard to talk these victims into believing that he could nullify the Kahuna's curse, but no one ever believed him, and so all of them died.

One day a Portuguese rancher complained to Dad that two thieves were stealing his cows. His cowboys knew who the thieves were, but they would not testify in court against them because a Kahuna, hired by the thieves, had told the cowboys that if they testified he would kill them.

My father said, "That's easy; just pay the Kahuna a bit more to pray the thieves to death." And the rancher said, "Why didn't I think of that?" Ten days later he returned to tell Dad that the thieves were dead, and it had cost him only "a cow and two pigs!"

In those days, there were no electric power lines in our village, so we had no access to any modern electric apparatus. In the evenings we used kerosene lamps. We had an old-fashioned telephone which was attached to the wall. When we "rang up," every curious person on the line could pick up his phone and listen to our conversation! Mail came every other day to an office about a mile from our home, and so I would walk there to pick it up. I had to watch carefully to avoid an angry bull that would sometimes come running along the narrow road trying to kill me! Once I avoided the bull only by beating him to the fence and rolling under it to safety. Another time the bull actually managed to toss me, but I fell into a river and so was not hurt.

My father was much handicapped by the absence of the wonderful drugs we have today. I recall once when my father operated to clean up the smashed hand of a fisherman who had held on to his dynamite too long. The operation was performed outside in our yard on the kitchen table. The Hawaiian minister gave the ether under my father's direction. After the operation, the patient just got up off the table and walked home with some friends!

Dad informed me that in years past a doctor might be trained not in college, but by a doctor who would take the young fellow around with him on his rounds. Once such a doctor, upon seeing an elderly woman sick in bed, scolded her for drinking too much of a patent medicine that contained a significant amount of alcohol. When the two men got back in the buggy the lad asked the doctor, "How did you know that woman was drinking too much of that patent medicine?" And the doctor replied, "I knew because I looked under the bed and saw many bottles of it." At the next stop the doctor said, "In this case *you* tell *me* what is wrong." The patient was a young woman.

The young doctor scolded her for carrying on an affair with the minister. On leaving, the doctor inquired., "How did you know that she was having an affair with the minister?" And the lad said, "I did like you did; I looked under the bed, and there was the minister!"

I profited from the education my father gave me, but I also exulted in the beauty of Nature all about me, and in the love and affection I received from my parents. When I was eighteen or nineteen I climbed to the top of Kaala, a nearby mountain with an altitude of nearly 4,000 feet. I saw the old volcanic crater filled with muddy water and moss-covered trees and I remember my wonder at seeing for the first time the remarkable plant with huge leaves called the *apeh apeh.* Later I also found it growing on the north slope of Haleakala, the huge extinct volcanic crater on the isle of Maui.

Because there was only an Hawaiian school in Waialua, for some 12 years my education suffered. Fortunately, my father taught me much as we drove around in his buggy. I learned not only English, geography, and history, but also the Greek and Latin roots of many terms used in science.

In 1895, out of all the doctors in the Islands, my father was chosen to try to find a cure for the many lepers in the colony on the island of Molokai. This happy circumstance took the Alvarez family out of our lonely village and into the city of Honolulu. There — at last — I was able to go to school and have the run of a fine library.

CHAPTER III

1895-1901

In late 1895 my father, appointed by the Hawaiian Board of Health to hunt for a cure for leprosy, left Hawaii to study bacteriology in Baltimore, while my mother and we five children remained in Honolulu. That city was a joy to me. The first thing I did on arriving in Honolulu was to go to the library and take out a book. I was immediately entered in a private school run by two old French maiden ladies, but after some months, disgusted with their poor teaching, I managed to get my mother to take me out.

Mother then took me to the Honolulu High School which was housed in a beautiful old palace, once owned by a Hawaiian princess and her banker husband. There, the Dean, dear old Mr. Scott, put me into the second half of the highest grammar school year. Finding myself with a good teacher, I was happy.

After four months I was put into the excellent high school situated in the same building which housed the grammar school. My teachers were good, and I had four splendid year of studying Latin, French, physics, chemistry and mathematics. I graduated summa cum laude, at the head of my class. Much of my education came from reading many splendid books on geology, paleontology, evolution, Darwinism, and the islands of the Pacific Ocean.

Luckily I soon became the pet of the chief librarian, Miss Burbank, and before long I was the collector of the dues of businessmen who helped to support the library. Also, for a while I was in charge of the place during the dinner hour. It was a joy to me to have free access to

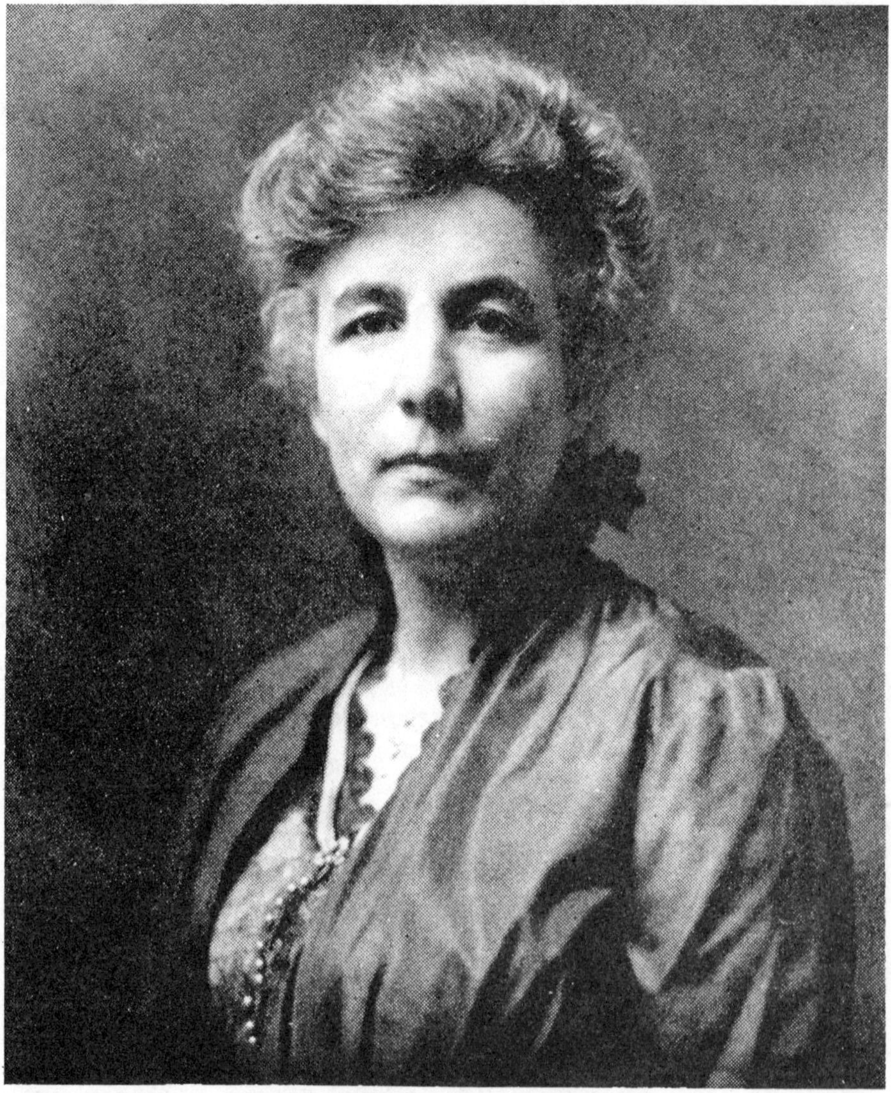

My mother, Clementina

the books that I loved so much.

Strangely enough, although during the eight years in Waialua I often went into the ocean or rivers with my father, I cannot recall his ever teaching me to swim. Shortly after I went to Honolulu, I rambled down to the harbor and stood on the edge of a high wharf. A tough-looking man asked me if I could swim, and when I told him I couldn't, he grabbed me and threw me into the water! I didn't fear the water and managed to paddle many yards to a place where I could get out to the beach. Thereafter, when school let out, my pal Percy and I would usually jump on our bicycles and go to the club house on the eastern edge of the harbor where we would swim.

On many afternoons, after swimming, I would go to the Y.M.C.A. gymnasium where a gymnast who had once been a circus athlete taught me to perform well on the horizontal bar. I became an excellent handball player and the best quarter-mile runner and best high jumper in school. During the five years I lived in Honolulu I developed a good strong body which enables me still to walk about easily. Most of the strong muscles — which I still have — were strengthened not only in my boyhood but also during my college years, when I spent several hours every week in a gymnasium. Up to the age of forty-five I continued to do a lot of mountain climbing, having gone on a dozen month-long hiking trips into the high Sierras with the Sierra Club.

A year or so before I left Honolulu, my chum and I built a catamaran, which gave us a great deal of fun in sailing it. One day when my chum and I were swimming in the shallow ocean to the east of Diamond Head, we saw the fins of two big sharks coming toward us. We beat the sharks to the beach, but a man swimming near us was not so fortunate and was caught by them. I later saw an old Hawaiian fisherman catch one of the sharks and cut open its abdomen: there in its stomach was one leg of the man!

One evening, about 1899, in Honolulu, I witnessed the Polynesian ceremony of walking barefoot on hot stones such as those used in pits for cooking food. A pit perhaps twenty feet in diameter was first filled with burning wood and lumps of stone. Eventually the bottoms of the stones were red with heat, while the tops were black. Then a Tahitian priest, with bare feet, walked out over the rocks, supposedly protected by his god. My hunch that the tops of the stones were not very hot was soon confirmed when two American soldiers took off their shoes and stockings and walked comfortably over the stones!

In 1901, when I graduated from high school, my father took me to lunch at the Royal Hawaiian Hotel. When we were done he asked what I was going to do now. And I replied, "I am going to study to be a physician, am I not?" That pleased Dad very much, and it was not long before he took me on a steamer to San Francisco. There he arraged for me to live with Dr. Rigdon, an old college friend of his. He then got me accepted at Cooper Medical College (now part of Stanford University).

CHAPTER IV

1901-1905

In September, 1901, my father and I sailed for San Francisco where I was matriculated in what was then Cooper Medical College, but is now the medical department of Stanford University. In those days there were few medical schools in the country which required of their matriculants a pre-medical course, so my father thought I might as well go from high school directly into the professional college, and that is what I did.

Actually, I doubt if the lack of a pre-medical course handicapped me much; I easily made up for it later by reading many serious books. In my years in a research laboratory, whenever I wanted some special information in regard to some phase of modern chemistry, physics, biology, statistics, or genetics, I read rapidly on the subject, and soon learned what I needed to know. An educator might be interested in the fact that the pre-medical studies which are hard and dull for many students, were fun for me *when I needed them,* because I so greatly wanted the information I sought.

Many a student starting out in medicine asks me if, in order to succeed in life, he should graduate from a big-name school, and I say, "No." I have never felt any handicap because I got my basic training in a small "proprietary" school. If a man studies hard in college, and particularly if he does an outstanding job in his years as intern, resident, and graduate student, no one will care a hoot where he started, and certainly no patient will ever bother to examine his diploma.

When I went to college I knew that I was preparing myself for my lifework, and hence I buckled down and studied hard. Sometimes I said to myself, "Some day you may be in a lonely shack somewhere in the country, fighting to save the life of a young woman in a hard labor; or the life of a cowboy kicked in the head by a horse, and if then there is no other physician within miles who can come to help you, your patient's life will depend on your knowledge and skill."

Throughout all of my four years at college, I would go down town to the YMCA gymnasium three nights a week where I would spend half an hour on the mats with the wrestlers, then another half-hour teaching a squad either simple tumbling or the simpler stunts on the horizontal bar. After this, I would race rapidly back and forth a few times in the swimming-pool, and would then go home to study until about 10:30. Putting on light tennis shoes, I would then run a mile or more along the quiet streets to Golden Gate Park and back. In this way I kept my "wind" in good condition for an occasional quarter-mile race. Each day was very full of lectures and studies.

On Saturday evenings, with the two chums with whom I lived, I often went to theater. We sat in the top gallery where the cost was usually either 10 or 25 cents. Because we could run up 6 or 7 flights of stairs and knew exactly where to go, we generally got to sit in the front row.

As I look back on my first year in San Francisco, I wonder that I, who was only 17 and away from home for the first time, never felt even a twinge of home-sickness. Fortunately, I have always been like that.

One of my first disillusionments came when, at the age of 19, I discovered that even young men who were preparing themselves for their professions could not be trusted to behave sensibly and to *their own advantage.* Today, of course, this observation would not surprise me in the least.

When at the hospital I started as a clinical clerk, I was so delighted with the new experience that I jumped into the work with enthusiasm, and each week studied as many patients as I could. But then came a committee of my classmates to say that the laziest men in the class had decided that a patient a week was all they were going to "work up." If I were to go on preparing several cases a week, the professors would get ideas in their heads, and hence I was to "pipe down." I just went ahead with my work.

In 1905, when I became an intern, again I ran into the "slow-down;" and again I marvelled that so few of my fellows cared to take advantage of the good courses of training our teachers were offering us. Later, after 1926, when I had been teaching graduate students for years, I was again saddened to find some men trying to avoid working up more than a few cases a day.

Because I studied so hard during my first six years of medical training, I had almost no social life, but I felt no need of any. I took Osler's advice and kept my affections pretty much in cold storage. Every other Sunday I would cross the Bay to Berkeley to call on the young lady, Harriet Smyth, who, in 1907 became my wife.

Even before my intern year, I had gotten sense enough to be dissatisfied with a number of my teachers because they were not observers or thinkers, but just "givers-out" of what they had read in books. I cannot remember that any one of them ever thought of learning medicine from patients as I already was doing with my little note book.

I remember asking my old professor why a man in our ward who evidently was suffering from locomotor ataxia lacked much of the textbook clinical picture of the disease. When I asked, "How does it come about that some people have such an atypical form of their illness?" my Chief put his hand kindly on my shoulder and, with a twinkle in his eye, said, "Alvarez: remember this: *the Good Lord just won't read Osler!"* In other words, he told me not to expect all my patients to present *all* of the disease picture that is described in the textbooks. I am now interested to see that, so early in my life, I saw what, centuries before, the great Leonardo da Vinci had seen, that experience "is more truthful than books" — it is "the instructor of instructors." I saw what I was learning from books might be wrong, but what I was learning from listening to 100 patients was sure to be right.

Osler used to say that the doctor who does not study books is like a sailor who goes to sea without a chart, while the doctor who studies only what is in the books is like a sailor who so loves charts that he never puts out to sea! I have tried to be like a sailor who, though well supplied with charts, spends his life at sea, and there, for all his days, keeps studying the ocean around him — in all its moods.

During my first two long vacations from College I went to Hawaii and enjoyed being with my family, and visiting old school friends.

In my third long vacation I went to visit with my family then living in Cananea, Sonora, Mexico. There I worked for a big mining company, moving Mexican miners from a very unhealthy canyon up onto a good mountain side. During this time, my father helped me to perfect my knowledge of Spanish.

While a student "clinical clerk," I began to accumulate interesting stories of patients. I remember a man who was so extremely irritable that I remarked on it. He said "Yes, doctor, I am so damned irritable that sometimes when I wake in the morning I slap my wife's face, and I say, "There, that's for nuthin'; now you just try and start somethin'.' " Ever since then, whenever I gave my wife a present which wasn't for Christmas, or a birthday, or an anniversary, I laughed and said, "There, that's just for nuthin' " — and that was a little joke between us.

CHAPTER V

1905-1906

William Osler has always been my hero, my great teacher and my inspiration. In 1905, I bought his *Aequanimitas and Other Addresses,* a book which was to have a great influence on my life. Osler reenforced in me the idea that "medicine is an art, not a trade; a calling, not a business." As he said, "Often the best part of your work will have nothing to do with potions and powders, but with the exercise of an influence of the strong upon the weak; of the righteous upon the wicked, of the wise upon the foolish." In an old diary for January 23, 1906, I find a note showing that I was already wondering how I could so work and grow mentally and spiritually as to be of the most use *to humanity and to my profession.*

Osler impressed on his students the idea that their college education had been only a start — a beginning. In college a man should learn where to go in the library to find the information he needs. A physician worth his salt will keep studying hard all his days. "The all-important thing is to get a relish for the good company of the race in a daily intercourse with some of the great minds of all ages." "Many of you (doctors to be) will need a strong leaven to raise you above the dough in which it will be your lot to labour."

I learned from Osler that a fine physician should be a well-educated man, with much knowledge, not only of medicine, but also of general literature and the psychology of men and women. I was cheered by his statement that all doors will open to a man with the "Masterword, which is Work." I profited from his statement that everyone should live his life in "day-tight compartments," neither grieving over the mistakes of the past nor worrying about the problems of the morrow.

I have always believed strongly in Osler's injunction that everyone should "burn his own smoke," by which he meant that no one should grouse and keep telling people about his discomforts. In my many years with the Sierra Club, I found that one of the most important of their unwritten laws was that no one should ever even remark to his neighbor that it was raining, that he was wet and cold and hungry, and that dinner was late.

I was much influenced by Osler's chapter on the joys of collecting the old medical books that are classics. This idea of his started me on a hobby that is still giving me pleasure. During some 40 years I gathered a large library, and eventually I owned most of the books written by the founders of American Medicine. As I traveled around the country lecturing, it was my habit to spend much of my time between trains rummaging in old book stores, and many were the treasures that I picked up in this way.

Other hundreds of treasures were found by looking through the many catalogs of old book stores that each month came to me from all over the world. I have derived much of my education from these catalogs. They list books which have been good enough to survive 50 or 100 years. I am convinced that any man who hopes to be not only a leader in his specialty, but a good and interesting teacher, lecturer, and perhaps editor, should know well the *history* of his subject's development.

I liked Osler's idea that a physician should so live that, eventually, he will become a philosopher. In many ways I soon did become a philosopher — each day helping some of my patients with their life-problems. Also, I learned from Osler the great value of imperturbability to a physician, by which he meant the ability to stay calm, cool, courageous and resourceful, even in the presence of great turmoil, and perhaps acute danger to the patient before him. It is a quality that is greatly appreciated by people, especially when things are going badly — as when the head of a family lies very ill after a stroke or a heart attack or a hemorrhage. The physician who, in such a situation, shows signs of bewilderment, indecision, fear, or mental paralysis, will not meet the needs of the patient and his family.

Once in my childhood, I was impressed by signs of this imperturbability in the behavior of my father. As we were eating breakfast, a man galloped up on a lathered horse. Hurrying in, he said, "Doctor, get to my house as fast as you can; my wife is dying; you know where I live?" "Yes," said my father, "I'll get there as soon as I can," and with that, the man rode off. My father called the yard man; told him to harness the horse, and then sat down and finished his breakfast. Then, seeing that the buggy was not yet at the door, he started changing some things from one little black bag to another.

Finally, my tense and excitable mother, unable to stand Dad's slowness and calmness any longer, said "Oh, Lu, Lu, how can you keep puttering around with those bags? Didn't you hear the man say that his wife was dying? Why don't you hurry?" My father looked at her quietly and thoughtfully, and said, "Well, Clemmie, if the woman is really dying, I won't be able to stop her, and if she isn't dying, there is no hurry."

During my internship, I kept learning much about human nature, and some of the lessons I have never forgotten. One day in December, 1905, a prematurely-aged street-walker who was perhaps 30 but who looked 50, applied for admission. She wanted to spend the worst part of the cold and rainy winter off the streets and in the hospital. She was thin, scrawny and uncommunicative, and so afflicted with the diseases incident to her business that I became nauseated when I had to treat her. She had drunk rather heavily, and in order to stand her contacts with the rough men whom she kept picking up, she had been taking morphine.

I thought her a very poor specimen of humanity, and hence was puzzled when, a few weeks later, I saw that in the women's ward, she had become the nurses' pet; she had been given bed No. 1, next to the desk, and she had been made head pantry-woman. This was the most coveted position, because it gave authority and enabled the woman to get better food than was served to the other patients.

Wondering how the nice nurses could be so chummy with such an awful creature, I asked them what they saw in her.

They said, "Don't you say a word against Lizzie; she may never cop a prize in a beauty show or be a deaconess in a church, but she is a wonderfully fine person, and good clear through. You just come and watch her some night after twelve when, as often happens, all hell breaks loose, and the poor lone nurse who has to care for the upstairs ward as well as the downstairs one, is overwhelmed by the many calls made on her. Old Mrs. Murphy there in bed number 14 will wake and start keening over her boy who died years ago; then that foul-mouthed woman in number 16 will start cursing and yelling for a shot of morphine; that old woman in number 24, who is in her second childhood, will get up out of bed and start walking up and down the ward without anything on; that half-crazy one in number 8, in a nightmare, will start screaming that someone is cutting her throat; and then a dozen women will wake up and all will start calling for something or other.

"You'd think that some of the women who aren't very ill would get up and help the poor nurse, but, no; they just pull the bedclothes over their heads and try to ride out the storm. But not Lizzie; she always gets right up and goes to work. With Mrs. Murphy she is gentle and kind; she brushes her hair for a minute and sings her a little Irish song, and soon Mrs. Murphy is quiet. In some secret way of her own she scares the daylights out of that demanding old devil in number 16, and shuts her right up. With those who are really suffering she has a remarkably kind and soothing way. To one she brings a glass of water; to another she takes an aspirin tablet; to another a needed bedpan; to another, with cramps in her legs, she will give a bit of rubbing with magic hands. Usually, within 40 minutes, the place is quiet again, and then after having given the nurse a cup of coffee, Lizzie goes back to her bed!"

I have never forgotten the lesson I learned that day. The terrible winds of adversity that had blown for years on Lizzie may have toughened her exterior and made her unattractive, but they had not changed materially the good, responsible, kind-hearted person who lived deep inside. The nurses had discovered that original Lizzie, and it was she whom they liked and respected, and accepted as a dear friend.

I learned from Lizzie what Jesus meant when He said, "There is nothing from without the man that going into him can defile him." I have always wondered what sort of woman Lizzie would have been if the good-for-nothing husband of her youth had not deserted her, and left her broken, drinking heavily, taking dope, selling her body for what little she could get, and hoping that the terrible life that she was leading would soon kill her.

One day a big husky laborer came into my ward with the complaint that he had a frog hopping about in his stomach. He said he had gone to many doctors, begging for help in getting rid of the frog, but they would not believe him; they just laughed. In my youthful ignorance I thought it would be easy to cure the fellow by giving him an emetic, and while he was vomiting, to drop a palmed frog into the basin. When my old professor saw what I was planning to do, he shook his head and said, "It won't work; you cannot cure a fellow like that; you'll only waste your time."

The only trouble was that next day he came back to say that I had been just 24 hours too late; the frog had spawned, and there were now a dozen little frogs hopping around in his stomach!

One day during the winter of 1905, when I was in charge of the receiving room, an old vagrant came in with lice crawling all over the outside of his coat and dropping off him by the dozen with each step he took. He begged me, for God's sake, to help him. He said he had gotten into his miserable state while living in boxcars where he couldn't bathe. He had no change of clothes, and hence he did not know how to get rid of the hundreds of insects which were eating him alive. His shoes were full of the dead bodies of hundreds of the cooties that he had trampled to death. He had applied at the City Emergency Hospital and other places for help but always had been quickly chased out into the street.

I had a hard time finding an orderly who would tackle the job of helping the man, but finally I induced one of the men from my ward — as a favor to me — to take the man out into the backyard, to undress him, to burn his clothes, and to sluice him off with a hose. Then we had to clip off the man's beard and every hair on his head and body. Down at the roots of the hair of his beard, the lice — two or three deep — were fighting to reach his skin! In a few days the fellow petered out and died, for no reason that we could determine, even at autopsy. In my medical lifetime, I have seen a few other vagrants with lice crawling on the outside of their clothes, but never did I see one whose awful state approached that of this unhappy man.

In the women's ward we always had some elderly woman with chronic ulcers on the inner surfaces of her legs, just above the ankles. Generally, we first "cleaned up" the ulcer; then we would cover it with skin grafts. One day when I had gotten an old woman's leg ulcers ready, I told her that, with her consent we would perform the little operation the next morning. After a while she called me and asked how long it would take for her to get well. When I said, "Probably two weeks," she said she did not want to have the work done. Puzzled, I asked her, "But, why? Are you afraid?" "No," she said, "It isn't that. Don't laugh at me, doctor, but after nursing these ulcers for 20 years, I could not lose them that sudden!"

I marvelled at her honesty in giving me the real reason behind the choice to keep her big sores. Often since then I have suspected that a patient with some ache of nervous origin was hanging on to it because he or she "couldn't lose it that sudden."

One day in the hospital I learned how much sympathy and understanding can help a patient. In my ward there was a sweet Irish girl of 19 who had a terrible tuberculosis of a hip. To drain this, a surgeon had made two big cuts through the girl's hip muscles and down deep into the joint. Every day I had to pack these incisions with gauze so that perhaps the wound would "heal up from the bottom." I dreaded the job because what I had to do caused the girl much pain. One day, on my return from a week-end vacation, I found her running a fever because the foul dressings had not been changed. When I asked the nurses why the girl had been neglected, they said she would not let any of the other interns touch her. When I asked her why, she said, "Because *you* are sorry when it hurts me, and when you are sorry, I can stand the pain."

One morning when my Chief arrived I startled him by saying we had a leper in the ward — an old Chinese with a chronic "punched-out" ulcer on the bottom of one foot. Suspecting immediately that this might be due to leprosy, I pulled up his pajamas and, sure enough there I saw some whitish patches, each surrounded by a narrow, dark ring. When I reached up to my lapel for a pin to see if the skin was without sensation (as it would be if the patches were leprous) the Chinese said, "No feel-'um; no feel-'um." With this, the diagnosis was made, and next day the poor fellow was taken to the local "pest house."

A year later my dear good friend, Dr. Robert Langley Porter, got me the job of taking care of this pest house. While I was there I saw a girl of 19 with a severe form of leprosy which had almost destroyed her eyes, and had caused some of her fingers and toes to drop off. She had a child by one of the orderlies; obviously the man was not very particular in the choice of a love-mate!

When I started work at the hospital, some of my chiefs fired me with enthusiasm for certain types of strenuous treatment, and as a result I often gave ice-water baths to the patients with typhoid fever, or mustard packs to the patients with pneumonia. And then, one day, a wise old nurse said to me, "You know what we girls think? We think you are just wearing those poor people out. Why not let them rest and sleep? That might do them more good." I thought a while, and said, "You're probably right; I know that if I were the patient, I would want to be left alone." After that I never pulled very sick people around in order to give them a lot of examinations and treatments; I trusted to the statement of my wise old Professor, Dr. J. O. Hirschfelder, who used to say that for many illnesses the best treatment is *"the blessed tincture of time!"*

One thing that soon perturbed me at the hospital was the tendency of a few of my Chiefs to alter the original record of a patient so it would agree better with their theories or prejudices or desires. This behavior reminded me of the exhortation that Mark Twain once gave a group or reporters. With his usual mixture of fun and wisdom, he said that always when a man is sent out by his editor to gather some information, he should record accurately and honestly the facts as he heard them or saw them. Later, he could distort these facts to his heart's content, or his editor could re-write them to suit his particular bias.

I have thought of this statement whenever I have seen a physician erasing something from a patient's record because he refused to believe the statement of fact, or refused to accept the implications of the fact, or wanted the record to support an idea he had. To illustrate: if a man in my ward died after treatment with the favorite drug regularly used by one of my Chiefs, he might say to me, "Don't file this case record for use in the paper I am planning to write because the man was too neurotic to be a suitable case for study." Usually, so far as I could see, there was no good basis for his having said this.

As a surgical intern, I hated to see one of my Chiefs being dishonest with himself. For instance, one day he crossed out my record of the fact that one of our patients had developed typical symptoms and signs of an acute new ulcer within a few days after the performance of a gastroenterostomy (a new opening out of the stomach designed to cure the original duodenal ulcer). The doctor, an eminent man, explained that he would not believe a word that that patient might say. But I could see no reason for distrusting the fellow, he seemed like a fine, honest man. I felt that what the patient had said should have been recorded in his history, exactly as he had said it. My impression was that my teacher's behavior was based purely on his great reluctance to admit that a gastroenterostomy was not a good operation for a young man with a duodenal ulcer. Actually, after some 25 years, the operation had to be given up except for a few special purposes.

Another time when I had recorded the fact that a mentally disturbed patient had told me that his brother, his mother, and his mother's sister were in mental hospitals, I was distressed when a Chief of mine, who would not permit me to mention the word "heredity" in his presence, came along and angrily crossed out the note that I had made.

One of my teachers of surgery used to rather amuse us interns because he seemed so unconscious of the fact that he was not honest with himself. To show what he would do: whenever at an operation he found the gallstones he had expected, he would dictate to his assistant: "a stone-containing gallbladder was removed in the usual way." But when, on failing to find stones in the gallbladder of a woman whose abdominal distress was due to a depression, he would dictate half a page telling of a slight milkiness of her gallbladder wall; a slight thickening of the wall; one little adhesion between the gallbladder and the duodenum; a little rounding and softening of the edge of the liver; an enlargement of the lymph node draining the gallbladder; or a little hardening of the head of the pancreas. After watching our Chief do this a number of times, we interns knew perfectly well that this was his odd way of sayng that he had opened a normal abdomen by mistake.

My feeling, even in those early days, was that if my teacher had been scrupulously honest with himself and with us — his assistants — he would have written "normal gallbladder," and let it go at that. The only objection to this would have been that such a written record would have left him open to legal attack if the patient had later wanted to sue him. At one hospital in which I worked in my youth, many an appendix was removed supposedly to cure the "vapors" of a neurotic woman. When it appeared normal to the pathologist who examined it with his microscope, he would write, "chronic appendicitis, grade I." He did this partly for legal reasons, and partly so that the surgeon would not have him fired.

When, in my twenty-first year, I was rotated into a surgical ward, I did one of the most useful things I have ever done: I was able to get many surgeons to stop their routine pre-operative purging of patients. I probably saved millions of people from needless suffering, and I suspect I saved some from death.

I became very curious about this problem which did not seem, in 1906, to be at all curious to my surgical teachers. It was obvious to me that the routine and often violent purging of pre-operative patients was wholly unnecessary. The fact that the *emergency* patients, who had to be operated on without benefit of purging, did better, had no gas pains, and recovered more quickly, indicated that the purging was more harmful than healing.

I asked our surgical nurses what they thought, and they all said that the non-purged patients always do better than do the purged ones. The nurses also said that they dreaded the stormy results of the routine purging on the fourth day after the operation.

My fine professor agreed with me and the nurses — to his great credit — that preparatory purging was not necessary. But when I asked him why he ordered it every day, he admitted that he did not know why; he did it simply because it was then the custom to do so.

I can imagine a European-trained physician having the horrors over the idea of an intern arguing this way with the leading surgeon in his college and his state, but my then Chief, Dr. Emmett Rixford, was a "big" man, and we were friends, and so he never became impatient with me or tried to shut me up.

Then I went to the library, and after weeks of reading, I discovered that the practice of purging patients before an operation was a remnant of the idea of many primitive peoples that when a lad is to face any ordeal, such as torture incident to his initiation into the tribe, he must be *prepared* by purgation, fasting, vigils, and abstention from sex. In ancient Greece, a philosopher who was to debate with a man from another "school" first purged himself with the violent drug hellebore. This was to rid himself of peccant (harmful) humors (supposedly important body fluids)."

In 1918 I published this evidence in a paper and soon many of the surgeons throughout the world gave in, and either quit preparatory purging of patients, or toned it down so as to make it less harmful, or they ordered only an enema. One day the then leading surgeon of Los Angeles told me how grateful he was to me because at last he had the answer to a question that for a long time had puzzled him — namely — why, when he operated on a famous movie queen did she always have a stormy post-operative course, while a "nobody" in the County Hospital, on whom he performed an emergency abdominal operation, was usually up and walking around in three or four days. With my evidence before him he saw that in his anxiety to get a good result with the movie queen he had purged her particularly thoroughly, whereas the other woman had not been "prepared" at all. Later, some of the abdominal surgeons who had done much operating in front-line hospitals during World War I, wrote to tell me how right I was — they said their operative patients (who rarely were prepared) did unusually well.

Incidentally, during my first six months in the hospital I expected to be a surgeon, because that was what my father wanted me to be. But when I got "rotated" into a surgical ward, I discovered that I had very little interest in surgery. What most impressed me was my great and constant desire to get back to my *medical* patients, and particularly to the problems of diagnosis, which fascinated me. Accordingly, I wrote my father that I was sorry to disappoint him, but I was going to be an internist. He accepted this decision of mine without any protest.

Ever since then I have been saying to medical students, "Don't worry about what specialty to follow; you are likely to find out which it is to be — when the time comes."

For months I had in my ward a sweet gray-haired old German tailor whom I came to like. He was dying of tuberculosis, and he was down to skin and bones. Because the tuberculosis had eaten into his voice box, every cough was torture to him. Finally, a day came when he started to die in earnest. He would stop breathing for a few moments and seem dead, but then he would take a deep breath and regain consciousness for a while. This went on for several days until the poor fellow, hardly able to stand the suffering any more, begged me to put him out of his misery.

That night I gave him a grain of codeine which I hoped would be enough to ease his pain so he could get some rest. Actually, he did *sleep all night,* and, as a result, he woke in the morning feeling like a new man. Because he had been conscious when I gave him his "shot," his gratitude to me was pathetic. After that I gave him a grain of codeine whenever he needed it to control his suffering, and as a result, he lived comfortably enough for several weeks. Then, suddenly, a big hemorrhage came and carried him off. This experience taught me a good lesson, which is that a sedative usually will not shorten a dying man's life, as his family so greatly fears it will. Actually, by lessening his pain, the drug will *lengthen* his life.

I had a number of good teachers, but the most brilliant of all was Dr. Emile Schmoll. I immediately saw that he was the ablest of my Chiefs, and so I made a special effort to "work up" his cases for him. As a result, we soon became friends. He loved what we doctors call the art of "snap diagnosis," and was keen at it. A snap diagnosis is one that is made with a shrewd glance at the patient, and perhaps a couple of questions. Schmoll would take me out into the great corridor of the hospital where, while he smoked a cigarette, he would keep asking me, "That man with the queer limp — what has he got?" And I had to learn to tell the disease at a glance. It was splendid training for me. One day he was disgusted because I could not tell him what was wrong with a man who, when he walked, rose on one foot and then swung the other leg through a big arc.

"What's the matter with you?" he roared. "He has a wooden leg!"

At this time, studying clinical laboratory work almost entirely on my own time and initiative, I had learned so much about it that I was given the job of teaching "lab work" to the senior medical students and the interns at Cooper College. During the ten months between July1906 and February 1907, I did this teaching of laboratory technique, some residency work, and a good deal of study in the X-ray department of an oculist clinic.

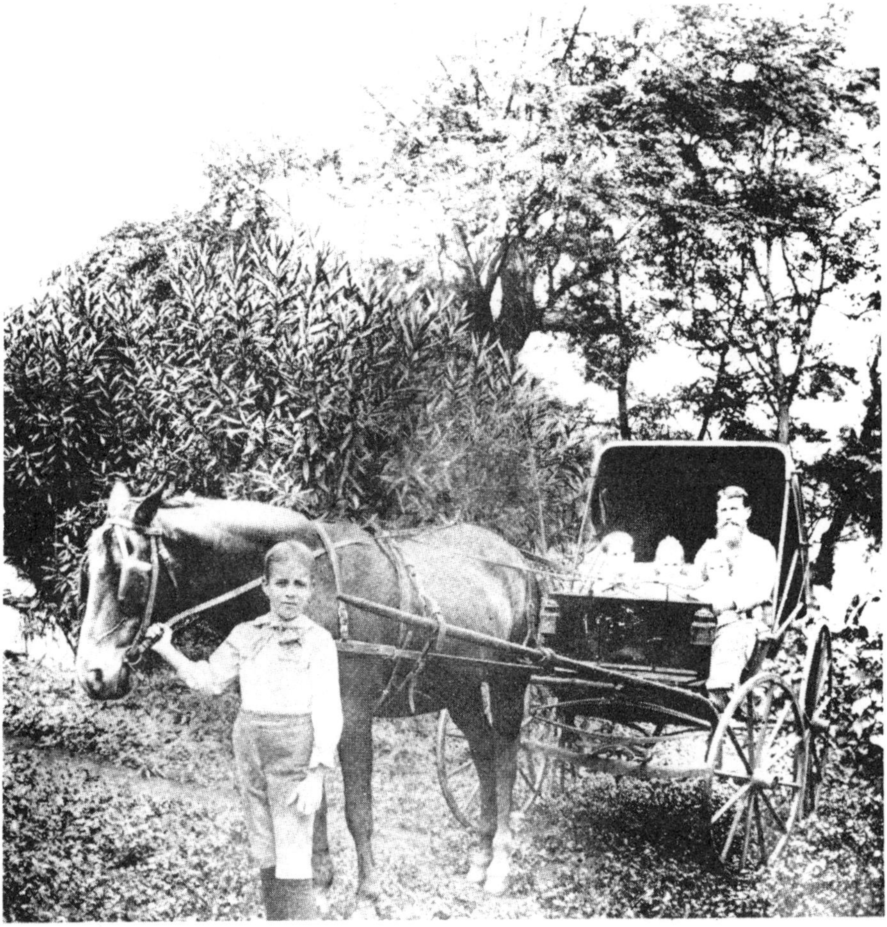

Taken about 1892, I am at the horse's head. Seated with my father — in his buggy, at Waialua are Milton, Florence, and Mabel.

CHAPTER VI

1907-1909

In February, 1907, when my father found that I wanted to get married to Harriet and to have a medical practice, he said, "Come and take over my practice in Cananea, I would like a long vacation, and perhaps even retirement." Actually he soon opened an office in Los Angeles, and practiced there until he died at the age of eighty-four.

Unfortunately, a week or so after my wife and I arrived in the big copper camp, the "bottom dropped out of copper;" the mines and smelters closed, and the wonder is that, with most the miners without an income, I had any practice. Fortunately, I made enough money to get by.

The poor people were so kind to me that I came to love them. I soon had a large obstetric practice; I saw many small children with diarrheas, and many women with hysteria. Because my college training in those three subjects had not been very good, I immediately bought books that helped me. I wondered if I ought to write the Dean of my old school and suggest that he give more and better lessons in neurology and psychiatry, and I wanted also to tell the professors not just to *tell* their students about nervous and mental diseases, but to *show* them patients with those diseases.

In 1907 if a nervous Mexican woman suffered some annoyance, she was likely to go into an "ataque" or attack, in which she would lie on her bed groaning or crying out, and having spasms in her arms and legs. In Cananea I saw many such spells of a type I cannot now remember having seen in the United States.

Fortunately, I immediately learned to stop these ataques by listening to the woman's heart with my stethoscope. If she kept crying out or struggling, I would say in Spanish, "Quiet down; how do you expect me to listen to your heart if you keep making so much noise?" All of the women I saw with ataques became quiet with this. The reason they were so glad to have me listen to their hearts was that they thought that some disease in the heart caused the "ataque."

Usually I gave the woman a sedative to keep her from starting up again; also I would tell the woman's mother to get all of the onlookers out of the room. Hysterical women have most fun when they have an audience. Some of the hysterical Mexican women whom I saw were in a trance from which I had to wake them. Some had false abdominal bloating due not to gas but to a contraction of the muscles lining the back of the abdomen. Some in a spell were so insensitive that they did not complain if a doctor passed a hatpin from one side of the thigh to the other. A few seemed to be paralyzed from the waist down.

In Mexico I learned so much about hysteria that years later, when I worked in the Mayo Clinic, I might recognize the disease the minute I saw a woman who was whispering, or limping in a peculiar way, or shuffling her feet, or walking with her body bent far over forward and turned so that she was looking upward.

In Mexico I saw a woman who lived in a house on top of a hill. One day lightning struck it, and the woman told me that a ball of fire came in, hit her right foot, and ran up to her groin, paralyzing her whole right leg. I took my small faradic battery with an electrode and said I would cure her by driving the lightning down and out of her leg. I stroked her leg, beginning at the groin and moving down to her foot and with this, she got up and walked, and was well.

Often I talked a hysterical woman out of her illness by getting her to face the fact that she would be much happier well; getting her to think of the possibility that if she stayed paralyzed too long, she might have trouble getting well. Several women said that they had worried about that possibility.

Once when I asked a hysterical elderly woman if her whispering was helpful to her, she said, "Yes, it keeps my vile-tempered old husband from snarling at me." 'All right then," said I, "I won't try to cure you," and we parted good friends.

A Mexican woman, with a contracted arm, did a strange thing. She travelled far to see me when she must have known that she got the contraction in order to punish her doctor after he had angered her. I quickly talked her into using the arm, but next day, when she came to say good-bye, she said she would keep it contracted a few days longer in order to punish her doctor some more.

Curiously, the first day when the woman came into my office, much worried and afraid, she had plenty of the vilest bad breath I had ever smelled coming from a human being. It stunk up my office so badly that I could not use the room until it had been aired for an hour. Next day when she was not worried or afraid of me, her breath was normal.

One of the most interesting patients I saw in Mexico was a big handsome man of fifty-five — sad-looking, haggard, and prematurely aged. He complained of panicky spells which deprived him of sleep. When I could not find anything physically wrong with his heart or other organs, I told him to call me the next time he had a spell, and I would go to his home to see him.

The next morning he called at 2 a.m., and I went to his house. There I was met at the gate by a big well-armed watchman who, after tying up two savage dogs, let me into the house. There I found the patient in bed, surrounded by guns. All that was wrong with him seemed to be a chill due to fright. I asked him what he was scared of, but he would not tell me, so I gave him a sedative and left.

A few days later I met an old prospector who told me that a year before, two Americans had found a fine copper mine. They had filed a claim but soon some men jumped it. The Americans sued to get it back, and the first judge awarded it to them, but a higher hudge gave it back to the thieves. The Americans sent a note to the superior judge saying that they would come back with guns and take him to the desert and fry him over a fire. That judge was my patient!

In Mexico I read not only much about gastroenterology, but much about psychiatry. I got started reading hundreds of books on mental troubles when in 1909 I bought and read Clifford Beers' great book, *A Mind That Found Itself* (1908). Beers was a Yale student, who, when his brother was stricken with what looked like epilepsy, soon got the idea that he too was getting it. That was in 1894. After graduation he went into business and did well. In March, 1900, after a severe attack of grippe, he went into a depression, and soon got the delusion that he was a hopeless epileptic. After nights of sleeplessness and thoughts of suicide, he jumped out of a window, and fortunately injured only his ankles. He lost contact with his relatives and became very suspicious of people because he was sure that by atternpting suicide he had broken a law, and could be executed for that; and because he thought everyone who spoke to him was a detective, gathering evidence for a trial, he would not speak to anyone.

If only a psychiatrist had thought of this fear, and had told him that he was safe from arrest because he had attempted suicide when he was insane, he could have been greatly helped.

Beers said so wisely that when he went insane, some of his senses began to play tricks on him, and to deceive him. For instance, when his food did not taste right, he thought it was poisoned.

As Beers said, certanly no one should get angry with a confused, insane man. That would be like punishing a child for having the mumps. When talking to an insane person one must always be kind and never contemptuous. Further, Beers said that he would have been a different man if he had been supplied with magazines and books; actually he was denied them by a stupid and vindictive doctor. Beers said that much reading matter could have helped him get well. There has been many a time in my office when, faced by a mildly insane patient, I have been so kind and friendly with him that he became friendly and trustful enough with me to take my advice — perhaps to see a good, able psychiatrist whom I knew.

Beers said that in his over-crowded and under-staffed hospital, no good treatment was given him. When he finally jeered at the stupidity of the doctor in charge, that man got so angry that he tied Beers up painfully in a strait jacket, and put him in the "violent ward" where he got beaten up and knocked down!

As Beers wrote later, "Never treat an insane man so nastily that he will get violent." After his four months in the violent ward, his brother put him in another mental hospital where an assistant was so kind to him that soon Beers became "good." He "didn't want to let the superintendent down." Beers got well when he was treated "as a gentleman."

When I read and studied Beers' book, I became so impressed with the helpful information I got from his book that I started buying and reading every such book I could find. After many years I had gathered some 850 such books, had studied them, and wrote a book based on them called, *Minds That Came Back.* I gave my "crazy library" to the splendid Mayo Clinic Library which for a period of twenty-five years had been such a great help to me. Later I found there is also a "crazy library" in the psychiatric department at Columbia University.

Late in 1909 I became desirous of getting back to a city — where I might perhaps have a teaching job in a medical school, and access to a big library and to book stores.

Then a miracle came: my favorite professor of my intern days, Dr. Schmoll, sent a note asking me to come to work with him.

As soon as my wife and I could pack up, we left for San Francisco.

CHAPTER VII

1910-1913

On January 2, 1910, I began work as assistant to Dr. Schmoll, a Swiss who had been very well trained in Europe under the great Dr. Naunyn. With Dr. Schmoll I was fortunate to have received special training in Internal Medicine.

During the first few months with the doctor, I spent most of my time taking histories, making examinations, performing laboratory and X-ray examinations and writing the requisite reports. I think it is interesting that had I not worked as hard as I did during my year of internship to become highly proficient in lab work, I could not have gotten this splendid job with Dr. Schmoll.

My Chief was a bachelor, about fifty years old. He was a tall, big man, a gourmet, a bon vivant with a talent for making interesting friends; but often he was so impatient and short-tempered that my friends wondered how I could get along with him.

I quickly learned to perform what was then the new Wasserman blood test for syphilis, and the money I earned for doing that work, for the patients of several physicians, added some much-needed income. On some mornings Dr. Schmoll and I worked together in a free clinic. In my spare time I studied gastroenterology in the splendid Lane Medical Library.

Because my Chief hated to write letters, I made our large consultant practice possible by writing the reports of patients' examinations and sending them to the referring doctors. Soon I had to go even further — writing Dr. Schmoll's love letters!

I remember well the first one I wrote. A gushing divorcee of 40 or so — a patient of ours — who evidently thought it might be a good idea to pick up a wealthy bachelor, wrote my Chief a "come on" letter. Dr. S. glanced at it, and gave it to me saying, "You answer it."

"But what sort of a letter should I write?"

So, imitating my Chief's handwriting, I wrote her a mildly affectionate letter.

Back came a perfumed missive saying, "Oh, Dr. Schmoll, you don't know how happy you have made me. To think that you, a great big man, should have stopped in your terribly busy day to write such a sweet sweet letter to poor little me has filled my heart with joy (etc., etc.)"

I have often smiled as I thought of that correspondence — wondering just how angry the lady would have been if she ever learned that I had written the letters that had warmed her heart. She came to the office a few times to see what she could do in the way of ensnaring my Chief, but he was wary, and saw to it that he was always so busy that I had to take care of her. With this, she gave up and quit coming.

Another handsome woman did much better with a simple approach; she just remarked to my Chief, "Five hundred dollars a month would keep me very comfortably!"

My three years with Dr. Schmoll was a time of great mental growth. I worked hard to add much to my knowledge of laboratory diagnosis; I kept reading and rereading Wood's big textbook on the subject until it fell to pieces in my hands. I had to work hard also to keep up with the big advances then being made in X-ray work. I had to make films of the teeth, which, in the beginning, without specialized apparatus, was a very difficult job. In those days I had even to cut and wrap the little dental films, because no company was as yet selling them.

From my Chief I learned a great deal about the then-new science of dietetics, and soon I was calculating the caloric and other values of diets. Dr. Schmoll was one of the first men in the United States to reduce people's weight with a scientifically designed low-calorie diet. The idea was so novel that one day a not overly-bright society woman made the mistake of thinking that the diet was like a bottle of medicine, to be added to her regular diet! When, after a week, she came in weighing several pounds *more* than before, Dr. Schmoll roared, "You *must have eaten* more than the food I prescribed"; and the woman said, "Of course, I have also eaten my regular meals!" This story so amused the woman's relatives and friends that it quickly spread all over the country.

Dr. Schmoll was the most brilliant "snap diagnostician" I have ever known. I remember the day a man came in and Schmoll, noting a glass eye, asked, "Was that eye removed for a little black tumor?"

"Yes," said the man.

"Now you have pains all over?"

"Yes."

Turning to me, Schmoll whispered, "Black cancer all over him."

And he was right. The man was soon dead.

One day a boy came in with his mother, and Dr. Schmoll remarked to her, "You nearly died in labor with that boy."

"Why, yes," said the woman, "but how could you possibly know that?"

Turning to me he said, "Look at that unusually deep, old forceps scar over his left eye."

One day Dr. Schmoll said to a patient, "You have polyps (small, soft nodules) in your nose, and chronic asthma; and for years you have been dropping a blackish silver-containing drug into your nose."

The man, astonished, said, "Goodness gracious, you're right!"

Schmoll said to me, "Look at the wide bridge to his nose, listen to his nasal voice, look at his bluish skin (filled with silver from the drug); note his barrel-shaped chest, his 'spade-shaped' finger-ends, and his contracted neck muscles in front — all signs of an old asthma."

One day a woman came in and instantly my Chief said, "Old exophthalmic goiter, and still a fibrillating heart." (A fibrillating heart is one in which, in the auricles — the two small chambers at the top of the heart — the muscle is not contracting as a unit, but each fiber is quivering separately.) Such fibrillating is common in cases of long-lasting toxic goiter. When I was puzzled, Dr. Schmoll said, "Look at that scar of a goiter operation peeping out from under her string of pearls, look at those shiny, rather frightened eyes, also, note her dark reddish skin, that tremor of her hands, and that irregularly irregular pulse in the side of her neck." It was irregularly irregular because the fibrillating auricles at the top of her heart were not supplying the ventricles (big pumping cavities) with the regular beat.

Dr. Schmoll was always doing that sort of thing. When walking out to luncheon with me, or while seated in the restaurant, he would say, "Look to your left and see the woman with myxedema (marked by a puffy, dull-looking face due to a loss of function in the thyroid gland). Or he might say, "Look at that man, he once had a Bell's palsy (paralysis of half of his face);" or "Look at that pale-skinned man who has either pernicious anemia or a severe form of kidney disease."

After a while I began to try my hand at this sort of diagnosis, and when occasionally, I "hit the bull's-eye," I derived great pleasure from the practice of the art.

One day I found in my office a friendly old fellow whose complaint was that he was "too tired even to go fishing." He had been thoroughly examined by three able physicians who, when they could not make a diagnosis, asked me to see him. Following in the footsteps of my Chief, I just said to the man, "On this hot July day, what are you doing with those big winter galoshes on your feet?" And he said, "Oh, doctor, I am so cold." Because he did not have the pudgy look of most persons with a complete loss of function of the thyroid gland, my able friends had failed to think of myxedema. Because they hadn't noticed his galoshes or thought of what his wearing them should mean, they had failed to make a ridiculously easy diagnosis. When I gave the old fellow big doses of thyroid substance, he quickly perked up, warmed up, and felt fine.

A snap diagnosis that surprised even me was one I made one day when called in consultation to see a woman of 35 with some curious distresses for which a thorough examination had shown no cause. The impression I gained from my first glance at her was so strong that I took a big chance and said to her physicians, "She has a tumor of the pituitary (the very important growth-stimulating gland at the base of the brain)." Because my friends were incredulous, I said, "Let's go to the X-ray room and get a lateral film of the head." When the film was lifted out of the clearing solution, there, sure enough, at the base of her skull was a *sella turcica* (the bony "Turkish saddle") much distended by a pituitary tumor.

The doctors then all said at once, "But, Al, how did you do it?" What had struck me forcibly was that this small woman had the big forearms of an athletic man — something I had never noticed before. Usually, a pituitary tumor produces a big nose, a big lower jaw, big hands and feet, and perhaps a raucous voice, but in the case of this woman, the excess of growth hormone coming from the gland had made only one big change in her, and this was in her forearms.

The fanciest bit of snap diagnosing I ever attempted was done just as a stunt to show some graduate students what can sometimes be accomplished. The X-ray man chose a chest film full of abnormalities. I was able to guess that the roentgenogram was that of a woman about 50, rather tall and thin, frail, and a Catholic. She had had several children. In her youth she had some tuberculosis, and possibly a mild polio. She once had a pneumonia with empyema. She could have been thrown once from her horse. She probably had a moderately high blood pressure with some arteriosclerosis, and she had suffered at times from arthritis. She used sometimes to go out with a brother or husband to shoot pheasants.

How could I guess so much — and so much that happened to be correct? I explained. The thin bones and the size of the breasts showed that the film was that of a woman. The fact that the breasts were hanging down suggested that she had had several children. The marked calcification (filling with lime) of the rib cartilages in front suggested she was over 45 and frail. (Such frailness with calcification has been shown in statistical studies.) The length of the thorax showed she was tall and thin, and the narrow "coatal angle" made by the ribs and cartilages as they spread out from the lower end of her breastbone, suggested again that she was often sickly (also shown statistically). The medal on a chain around her neck indicated Catholicism. Calcified scars in the lungs and on the side of the neck showed that she had had tuberculosis. One arm a little smaller than the other suggested an old polio. A scar on one rib, marking where a tube had gone in for the drainage of pus, showed she probably had had a pneumonia with subsequent empyema. A healed fracture of the collarbone suggested a fall from a horse. The somewhat enlarged left ventricle (large pumping chamber) of the heart suggested a high blood pressure, and a calcification of the arch of the aorta — the big artery which comes out of the heart — suggested a tendency to hardening of her arteries. A marked roughening of several of the vertebrae where the ribs joined the spine, showed a tendency to arthritis, and three birdshot in the muscles of one shoulder suggested a hunting accident.

During my years with Dr. Schmoll, I kept constantly learning medicine — some of it from books and journals, but much from my daily study of symptoms as they appeared in people. At the end of each year I would sum up in my diary the new skills I had acquired, and usually then I would marvel at all the facts that a young physician must store away in his mind if he is to be a good diagnostician, a good physician, a good teacher, and a good consultant.

In 1912 a favorite "fashionable diagnosis" was "intestinal autointoxication." When a nervous woman felt tired and toxic and below par, and suffered from headaches, she was likely to be told that she was absorbing poisons from foul material in her large bowel. This explanation sounded so reasonable that most persons were well satisfied with it. But I always doubted if it was correct, and one day I knew it was *not* correct.

That day, after luncheon, my Chief came in looking the picture of dejection and misery. He said that because of a blinding headache he was going home and to bed, and I was to take care of the patients as best I could. A few minutes later I heard him out in the hall whistling merrily as he walked back to the office. He came into my room and said, "After I left you a few minutes ago, it occurred to me that because of an emergency call early this morning I forgot to do what I always do. So I went and attended to the matter; and now, here is the astonishing observation. *Before I left the men's room* my headache was gone, together with my feeling of depression and my indigestion. I was trained as a biologic chemist and I am sure there is no poison that could have been removed from my blood that quickly. Evidently what was wrong was a depressing effect on my brain produced by the distention of nerves in the lower end of my bowel."

I agreed with my Chief, and told him that I myself had had many similar experiences in which I had obtained immediate relief from abdominal distress and headache, just as he had.

This conversation started me on a series of studies in which I soon showed that some highly sensitive persons could develop the symptoms of "autointoxication" when the end of their bowel was packed *with cotton!* This proved that the distress in the head could be due purely to pressure on the nerves in the rectum — if the person was *sensitive enough.* No such distress is produced quickly by constipation in the case of the average, somewhat insensitive person.

I showed next that in the case of constipation, in certain persons, symptoms such as hiccup, belching, gurgles running up the gullet, a feeling of pressure up against the midriff, a little nausea, flatulence, a feeling of abdominal distress, and even abdominal pain, can all be due to ripples starting in the distended and hence stimulated segment of bowel, and running back up the digestive tract to the throat. Whenever I have been constipated, and these symptoms have distressed me, they have stopped the instant the constipation was overcome. Eventually, I gathered and wrote up so much evidence against the idea of "autointoxication" that most doctors stopped making this diagnosis.

All my life I have had a tendency, if time was available, to go on questioning a patient about his or her symptoms long after I was satisfied as to the diagnosis. Why? Because I wanted to learn all I could about the natural and biological history of the disease. I wanted to learn from the patient what were the triggers that brought on his attacks, or if he had learned any secret of avoiding his spells of acute illness, or of shortening them when they came, and each day I kept recording the information I obtained. I always carried a little loose-leaf notebook in my pocket, and with this I obtained the information which went into many of my scientific papers. Also, with it I learned much of what I now know about medicine. With the help of my notes I learned from many hundreds of patients when it pays a person to part with teeth, tonsils, an appendix, or a womb — and when it does not pay.

I became so interested in what is now called *psychosomatic medicine* that on November 12, 1912, before the San Francisco County Medical Society, I gave my first paper on the subject. The doctors were so pleased with the idea that they gave me an ovation. Ever since that day much of my time has been spent studying the influence of a disturbed mind on the body.

A good example of the type of nervous illness that has fascinated me ever since is to be found in the case of a young woman of 35, who came to me with a fever of 101°, which she had been running for four years, ever since her marriage. Because of the abdominal pain that accompanied it, she had had three surgical explorations of her abdomen. I was soon convinced that there was no disease in her abdomen. I found that all her discomfort was due to her indecision about getting a divorce. Her long-standing disease vanished when she finally left her husband.

I learned in those early years of my practice that a confession made to a physician can be just as effective in clearing the mind and body of distress as is a confession made to a priest. One day a very attractive woman of fifty had become so angry with Dr. Schmoll for dismissing her because he could not find a cause for her chronic abdominal pain that she refused to leave the office, In exasperation, he turned her over to me.

I asked her why she looked so unhappy, and after sizing me up for a moment, she said, "I believe that I can talk with you." She then proceeded to confess that in order to put her gifted son through an Eastern university, she had run a "call house" for four years. But when that job was done, she was overwhelmed with the conviction that she had become so foul that she disgusted people; she even felt that when she passed a group of people on the sidewalk, they would divide, separating themselves from her. I quickly assured her that she was mistaken, and told her that I admired her for what she had done. I felt that any son whose mother had run a house like that to put him through college should have adored her.

I got to talking with her about the problems she had with running the house. I wondered how she had handled the pimps and alcoholics, and if she had had a doctor to fight venereal diseases in her "girls." My secretary came in at that point and asked me if I could stop and take care of two patients who needed to return home soon, and if I could have this woman come back tomorrow. But the lady said, "No. Dismiss me now. I am cured!" "But how on earth could you be cured?" I asked. And she said, smiling at me, "Because you *like* me." There was no doubt that I did like her. The fact that a man in my social position was not disgusted with her satisfied her that she was not a social pariah, and she knew that she no longer had to feel literally "sick with shame." In much the same way, I have comforted thousands of worried and unhappy women, largely because I had compassion for them and made it clear to them that that was so.

In my "medical confessional," perhaps the most remarkable story I ever heard was that told me one day by a sad-looking woman of 45 who came to consult my Chief and me about her ill-health, her indigestion, her insomnia, and some pains here and there. After a thorough examination had failed to show anything physically wrong, I asked her why she was so unhappy. After crying a while, she said that many years before, a handsome lawyer had been trying for months to get her pretty but very selfish younger sister to marry him. When the sister finally told the man she would never accept him because he wasn't rich enough to suit her, he became so angry that he said to my patient, "Let's you and me *show her;* let's *us* get married." Because my patient really liked the man, and very much wanted to be married, she snapped him up.

After the wedding they went to his lodge for their honeymoon. A few days later the younger sister, having decided that she really wanted the man, came to the cottage to take him away. He was delighted with her idea, but not knowing exactly what to do with his bride he decided that, for a while, the two women would sleep together with him in his big bed! Finally, after twelve years of this, when my patient had become a nervous wreck, her sister decided she had had enough and left.

When I asked my patient why she had put up with the situation for so long, she said she was too weak-wiled ever to stand up against her domineering husband and her steely-hard sister. For the first few weeks she had wanted to hang on to her legal rights, and later, when she found she was pregnant, she felt she just had to stay on because she could not go out to face the world alone. When two more children came, she felt all the more that she would have to stay.

In 1912 my acquaintance with some mentally disturbed members of two distinguished families started me on a life-long study of the inheritance of equivalents of psychosis. In one family there was great ability in some of the members, but there were spells of insanity in one sister, another sister was a stout woman with a low degree of intelligence, another sister was a recluse who could not make up her mind about anything, and a brother had made a mess of his life.

In the other distinguished family that much interested me, the first person I saw was a woman of 30 who came to consult me about a mentally retarded daughter. When I noted that the woman herself was a bit psychotic, I asked her about her family. I found that she had a handsome and brilliant but asexual sister, and six big, fine-looking brothers, one of whom was a periodic drinker — a "lost week-ender." The father was a very able and much respected man, but his brother was a red-nosed, skid-row type of alcoholic.

Also at about this time I saw a quick-tempered man who looked to me like some epileptics I had seen. He complained of terrible headaches. I asked him if there was epilepsy in his family, and he told me that his brother was in the state epileptic colony. When I treated him as an epileptic, he got well! It was he who introduced me to the idea of carriers of epilepsy without seizures.

At a later time, when I was at the Mayo Clinic, I became interested in watching out for these people and I found about four hundred of them. Dr. Frederic Gibbs, that great encephalographer of Chicago, once told me that for every epileptic he saw with convulsions, he saw ten without. It is interesting to note that Professor Stanley Cobb of Harvard corroborated this.

In 1972, I wrote a book about 274 such seizureless epileptics *(Nerves In Collision)*. In it, I listed 250 references to articles concerning these mild epilepsies — but that did not keep many doctors from jeering at my "crazy theories." They failed to note that I had not written about "theories." I had written about 274 patients that I myself had seen and usually cured.

While practicing with Dr. Schmoll I began to notice something which I had not heard about in college — that many "chronic" complainers do no have any localized disease that can either be cured by medicine or removed by surgery. Many a person — and often a frail-looking one — seems to have been born to be uncomfortable, with "poor materials" built into his or her body. I sensed that many of these persons are doomed to live out their lives in weakness and frailty. Any cold or little infection can lay them low for weeks, and rarely can a physician make such a person over into a strong, robust and uncomplaining hard-worker. Many will have no stamina, and for all their days will complain bitterly about some scratch, little bruise or pimple. Many will always have the "habit of illness." When inducted into the Army, most men of this type promptly "crack up" and have to be sent home. It isn't their fault; it is the fault of an inherited frail body or troubled mind. These are the people who, as Osler once said, you will have to keep helping as long as they live.

I remember well a tall, thin, always tired and sickly young man of this type. My deep interest in his problem started me on a lifetime of study. His mother and sister were tall, thin, and frail, just like him. For a while his sister was mentally disturbed — and later I found that many constitutionally frail persons have psychotic relatives. Recently, I saw this old friend and patient of mine. He is now in his eighties — a thin gray-haired man — still frail and ailing. I take my hat off to him because he has always had the guts to keep earning his living. It is sad that he never felt strong enough to take on the responsibilities of marriage.

In my efforts to get a better understanding of this type of illness, I did much reading in physical anthropology and on the relation between physical build and mental capacity. I read everything I could find on fatigue. Eventually I came to the conclusion that constitutional inadequacy is more likely to be due to a peculiar brain than to a peculiar body. Some of these patients are highly intelligent and able, and some are well built, but they cannot stand up to much strain. In 1942, after two years spent in organizing my thoughts on this problem, and polishing

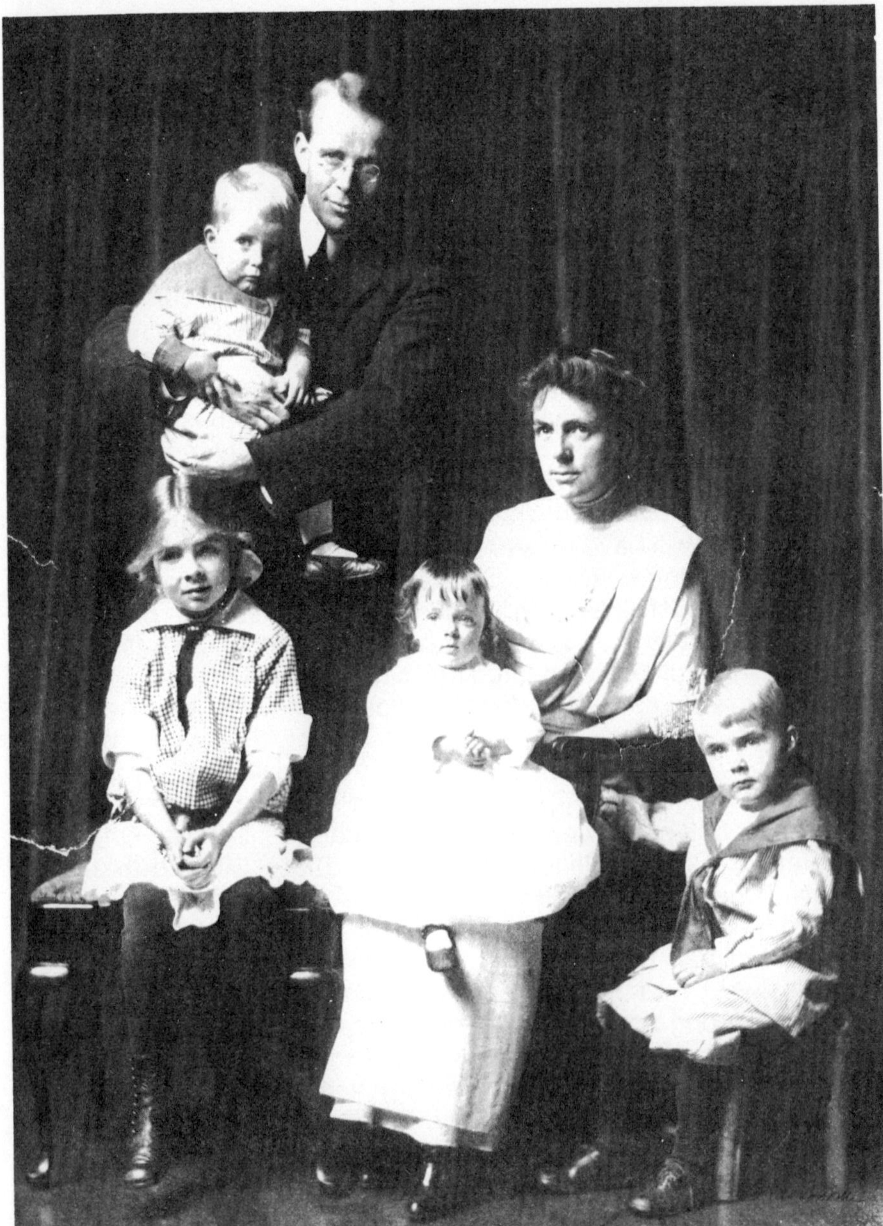

Our family: I'm holding Robert, and Bernice is on my wife, Harriet's, lap. Gladys is to the left of her mother, and Luis is on the little stool on the right.

and re-polishing a paper on inadequacy, I published it in the *Journal of the A.M.A.*

During my years with Dr. Schmoll I came to see ever more clearly that my interests were centering in the *diagnosis of chronic abdominal diseases.* I never was much interested in patients with *acute* illnesses, and when I was at the Mayo Clinic I never had a hospital service.

Because by 1913 I sensed that some day I was going to be a teacher of gastroenterology I started reading widely on the history of the subject. I wanted to know how knowledge had developed in this field of science, and who were the great pioneers. Also, I felt a need to read every article I could find in several languages on the minute structure and function of the digestive organs and the nerves that supply them. I did so well on this and on my researches in the "Gastro" field that in 1929 I became President of the American Gastroenterological Society.

I realized that if I were ever to be the sort of physician and teacher I wanted to be, I would have to learn to read rapidly in several languages. I already could read Spanish and French easily. I could understand medical Italian well enough, if only because I had studied Latin for four years. What I lacked was German; and so in 1912 I began to study this language. Many an evening I read German articles and books, with a teacher by my side to help me over rough spots. By 1916 I had become very proficient in medical German. A busy scientist must learn to "skim" and to read a paragraph at a time. I fear that no one who reads slowly and with difficulty can ever hope to gain an encyclopedic knowledge of his branch of medicine. He just won't have the time. A busy physician has only a few minutes a day for keeping up-to-date, and hence he must use this time for reading the best articles and chapters of books. Furthermore, most of his information must be derived from good abstracts or summaries of articles. Every month I read many book reviews in order to find the volume I should be reading.

I soon realized how fortunate a physician is when he can and will give his patients a clear and simple understanding of what he thinks their trouble is, or tells them what is hopeful about their condition, or what he plans or hopes to do in the way of treatment. Dr. Schmoll's words were so technical, his speech so thick and Germanic, and his patience so short, that few lay persons could learn much from talking to him. As a result, many of his patients, after leaving his office, would come around to my door and ask, "What did my examination show, and what did Dr. Schmoll think about me?" Then I would explain, in words of few syllables. In doing this I made many friends who later went out of their way to help me start my own practice in San Francisco.

Unfortunately, quite a few physicians today *pride themselves* on their ability to use long technical words. They will say "cerebrovascular accident" for a "stroke," and "urticarial wheals" for "hives." They make me think of the time in 1667 when Professor Christian Thomiseus of Leipzig had the temerity to lecture in German — instead of Latin — and for this was expelled from his university!

Nicholas Culpepper (1616-1654) similarly offended the Royal College of Physicians of England when he translated — from the Latin — the London Pharmacopoeia (the official list of drugs), and described these drugs in the English language.

I agree with Dr. William Bennett Bean that many physicians who write in a ponderous way, using long and obscure words, are fooling themselves into believing that they know a lot, when really they don't.

As "Boss" Kettering once reminded me, too often the explanation given by a teacher does not explain anything. One day in his youth Kettering was disturbed because his teacher seemed perfectly satisfied with the statement that we can see through glass "because it is transparent!" Young Kettering wanted to know what is peculiar about the arrangement of the atoms in glass that allows the waves of light to go through.

I always believed my Chief was wrong in thinking that by translating a patient's complaint into Greek, he had thrown a great light on it! When a psychotic girl came in weighing only 78 pounds — for months she had refused to eat — my Chief was satisfied when he said she had *anorexia nervosa*. But, young as I was, I saw that he had merely said *in Greek* that she had "a nervous lack of appetite." Because we doctors are so satisfied with the words *anorexia nervosa,* it is a rare physician who notices that many girls of this type are mild schizophrenics. But even the man who says the girl is "schizophrenic" has done little more than to express in Greek the recently popular, but probably meaningless, theory that the girl has a split personality!

I remember occasions when my Chief fooled himself in still another way. Once, a purblind and partially paralyzed young woman came in and we made the diagnosis of multiple sclerosis. Dr. Schmoll, like many other physicians, thought that having given a name to the disease, we could look in a book and see how to cure it. But, of course, we couldn't cure it. Even today, half a century later, no one can cure it.

It would be bad enough if we doctors just fooled our patients. What is sad is that so often we fool ourselves! As Osler used to say, it is bad for the doctor when he "can fool himself to his heart's content all the time." Early in my career I learned that even some able physicians can never do research of any value because, like many psychoanalysts today, they start their study with the conviction that they know what the answer is going to be.

My Chief used to give a woman a medicine and tell her to take it for a week, and then report. When she returned, he'd fix her with a menacing eye, and say, "You're much better, now don't you deny it!" Under these circumstances it was only a very courageous, or honest, or stubborn woman who would keep maintaining that her symptoms were unchanged. Obviously, any paper on a drug action that my Chief might write could not have much value. And yet, I am sure he had no idea that he was fooling himself. He was quite naive in the matter.

Ever since my years with Dr. Schmoll I have worked hard to write well and clearly — in simple English, and in short sentences. I am sorry to say that after half a century of writing, the job seems to be just as hard as it ever was. My only comfort is that the master of lovely prose — Robert Louis Stevenson — confessed shortly before he died that for him, writing was still as difficult as it had ever been.

Early in my life I realized that some skill in public speaking could be a tremendous asset to me. In those early days, practically all doctors droned along, reading their papers without paying any attention to the audience. Hoping to learn how to do better than this, I read a book on public speaking, and learned that what is essential is that the speaker have a strong desire to pass on to his audience some information which he feels is interesting and important; also he must *give it* with enthusiasm.

Then, one hot day in June, 1911, at a big medical meeting in Los Angeles, after hours of listening to doctors wo had been *reading* apathetically, I saw a man come up onto the platform — a man who obviously was filled with enthusiasm about a discovery he had made — and who was highly desirous that all of us share his interest. He had no paper; he just talked and showed us some charts. As was to be expected, even those of us who had been drowsing, sat up and watched and listened. The man was the late Dr. Francis Pottenger, the great expert on TB, who later became a good friend of mine. I immediately said to myself, "I am going to learn to talk like that, even if the effort nearly kills me." Since then I have always *talked* from a few notes in my hand, and I think usually with some vigor and enthusiasm.

In my early years I suffered terribly from stage fright. While at a meeting waiting for my turn to speak, I would be ill, my heart pounding, my body shaking. I became cured of this when I started lecturing to medical students. I then said to myself, "You darned fool; surely you know immensely more about this subject than those lads do, so why should you feel at all self-conscious before them?" With this, I lost all of my uneasiness, and it never came back.

I learned that when presenting facts, it is very helpful to present verbal pictures. As the Arabs say, "He is the best speaker who can turn his listeners' ears into eyes." To illustrate: many a physician, in giving a case report, will start out saying, "A man of 50, of normal weight, with a normal white count, a hemoglobin of 85 per cent, etc." — and his audience will drowse; but let him get up and say, "A vice-president of a big corporation got up clumsily out of his chair in the reception room and started to walk into my office with short, shuffling steps. He said he was 50, but he looked 70. He was so slowed-up, and there was so little animation in his face, that no one would have hired him to run a popcorn wagon. He talked thickly out of one side of his mouth. He had a little egg on his chin, and some gravy down the front of his coat! A few questions showed that he had had some 'little strokes.' "

A picture like that grabs the interest of one's listeners, and the mental picture of that patient tends to stay with them for years.

I am glad that in my early years in practice I learned to say often to patients and consultants, "I don't know what is wrong." This behavior was good for the development of my mind and character, and it made many friends for me. Osler taught that to say, "I don't know" is much better than to beat about the bush. Often an intelligent patient has said to me, "I like your courage and honesty in confessing your ignorance, and now I am going to stay with you until you say you know what is wrong. And then I'll believe you."

In my youthful days, when I had to deal with a millionaire, I was inclined to be awe-struck and ill-at-ease with him. But one night I was so well cured of this fear of the wealthy that I never suffered from it again. What happened was that, around midnight, my Chief asked me to make a call on one of the wealthiest of our California millionaires. I remember going up to the door of one of the biggest "palaces" that then lined Pacific Avenue. After I had rung for a while, the butler came over from the servants' house, took me up an imposing stairway, and then back through a long dark hallway to a great big, poorly-lit room.

There, all alone in a canopied bed, sat a little old man who I saw was "scared to death." He thought he was about to die with a heart attack, and he particularly dreaded dying all alone with no one to keep him company. As I remember, he had a wife and daughter, but they were in Europe. His son was playing polo somewhere. I wound up feeling so sorry for the lonely old fellow that I stayed for an hour trying to cheer him up. I hated to leave him alone again in that huge dark house.

In 1912 I became very interested in the news then coming out of Europe to the effect that, with a good roentgenoscope (X-ray screening apparatus used in a darkroom) one could watch the stomach and bowel at work, and could see a peptic ulcer or a cancer. Realizing how valuable such a technique could be, I talked Dr. Schmoll into going to Vienna so that he might study under the famous Dr. Holzknecht. Once that was accomplished, I managed to have him send me the large European vertical roentgenoscope.

But late in that year, any delight I had felt about the new instrument was over-shadowed by the unhappy changes in Dr. Schmoll. He became much more irascible and unreasonable than ever before. I am ashamed to say now that I did not then make the correct diagnosis of a begjnning psychosis. This man, who was destined in a few years to go insane, started out in life with a tendency to eccentricities. As a result, when he began to slip into a psychosis, all that his friends like me could see was a greater tendency to eccentricity.

During the very trying last four months of my life with Dr. Schmoll, I kept asking him if there was some tragedy in his personal life that was distressing him terribly and making him so irritable. But he kept answering that all the trouble was with me — that *I* "was going crazy!" Eventually, the strain of trying to keep the peace with him became too great, and I had to leave. Four years later he had to be committed; and much to my grief, it was in the asylum that he died. I have always regretted that I did not have the wisdom then to see what was happening to this once great physician.

On leaving Dr. Schmoll, I went to Boston (having left my wife and children in Berkeley with my mother-in-law) where I wanted to get answers from the great physiologist of Harvard, Dr. Walter B. Cannon. He was, I think, the first man in America to use the newly-discovered X-rays for studies of the movements of the digestive tract.

It was, I believe, in April, 1913 that I first went into Dr. Cannon's office. I found him to be very kind and friendly. I asked him ten questions, none of which he could answer. He then did a remarkable and generous thing: I was a stranger to him, and yet he said, "You are obviously so anxious to secure information that I suggest you go into my private laboratory in there and try to get for yourself the answers to the questions you have in mind." Dr. Cannon took me into the lab and showed me how to anesthetize a rabbit, and there to study its bowel under a bath of warm saline solution.

Right away I went to work studying flatulence, by seeing what happened to oxygen, carbon dioxide, and nitrogen when each was injected into the different parts of the small bowel. I was excited to find a very interesting gradient in reactivity in the small bowel, with a prompt reaction in the upper end, and a slower and lesser reactivity in the lower end. Then I found similar gradients in the sensitivity and rate of rhythmic contraction of resected segments of the bowel.

When I showed my findings to Dr. Cannon, he was delighted, and said that I had made such a valuable discovery that I must keep studying the gradients. He added that a similar discovery of gradients in the reactivity of the muscles of the heart had been of great value to medical science.

I did what Dr. Cannon advised, and for the next 17 years (until the financial crash of 1929, when I lost my laboratory), I spent my mornings studying the movements of the stomach and bowel, and writing and lecturing about my findings. Dr. Cannon helped me greatly by editing the text of my first physiological paper on the gradients.

Another splendid result of my trip to Harvard was that Dr. Cannon became one of my dearest friends. After I returned to San Francisco, we continued to correspond right up until his death. In fact, I've always been touched by the fact that Dr. Cannon wrote a letter to me the very day before he died.

He had a great sense of humor, which I loved. One morning when he came into the laboratory with a smile on his face, I asked him to tell me what had pleased him so. He said that he was happy because the evening before, his young son had shown that desire for accuracy and that willingness to repeat his work to get accuracy (which are signs of a scientific inclination), in a very humorous way. His son was at his mother's knee trying to recite the Lord's prayer, but he had made a mistake, and he said, "Now, damn it, I'll have to start all over again!"

Another time when Dr. Cannon looked downcast, I asked him why. He said, "Today, I feel like hiring someone to kick me around the block for trying to be a physiologist. Physiology is now mainly biochemistry — and I am no chemist. My main training was in biology. I feel as if I am being left so far behind in my own field of endeavor that perhaps I should quit trying to keep up."

"But Dr. Cannon," I said, "Surely you have done so much for physiology that you could even afford to lie abed all day for a while and let the other men catch up to you."

"No," he replied, "Someday, when you have many achievements to your credit, you will have learned that what you *have done* gives you little joy or comfort. It is only what you hope to do and plan to do that interests you."

And later I found that what he said was true. I have had over a thousand papers and many books published. But what interests me are works in progress, and future publications. It is the work ahead that matters.

In 1931, I was pleased and honored to have been chosen to represent all of Dr. Cannon's students in a speech given at Harvard for the celebration of the 25th anniversary of his professorate. Many eminent scientists and fine people were there, and that evening my wife and I were guests in Dr. Cannon's home.

My life was enriched by his friendship. One day I asked him what he grew on his farm in New Hampshire. With puckish humour he replied, "Stones and children!"

The corrrespondence between Dr. Cannon and me was extensive, and told a great deal about the advances in physiology in our day. I was thus gratified when Harvard requested — and received — our voluminous correspondence for their special library.

CHAPTER VIII

1913-1926

When in 1913 I returned from Boston to San Francisco, my savings were so nearly used up that I wondered how I could start practicing on a shoestring in a big city during those first two years when few people would know about me. But then there came a friend, Dr. Carl L. Hoag, an able young surgeon who worked mornings as assistant to the professor of surgery at the University of California.

Carl said he wanted to open an office in which he could work from two to four, and I could have the place from four until six. I gladly accepted his offer. As I had expected, for the next two and a half years my practice did not grow, and each month I took in just enough money to make ends meet.

Then, suddenly in December, 1915, many patients came, and soon I had to move into a bigger office where I had a secretary, a telephone girl, two laboratory girls, an X-ray girl, a part-time expert X-ray doctor, and a part-time doctor who took histories for me.

When I returned from Harvard, I greatly wanted to spend my mornings continuing with my physiological studies on the stomach and bowel, but for months I could not get much of a laboratory. But then a certain Mr. Hooper, upon dying, left a great deal of money for the purpose of establishing the Hooper Foundation at the University of California. This was housed in a large building full of laboratories situated on Parnassus Avenue in San Francisco. The Director was Dr. George Whipple, who with two assistants was studying the ability of the liver to influence the formation of the blood. He gave me a laboratory and an assistant; and as long as he lived he was my dear friend. For the next twelve years, until December 1925, I worked mornings at the Hooper Foundation. I published some forty papers during that time, documenting my work there. I became a member of a number of societies such as the American Physiological Association, the Society for Experimental Biology and Medicine, the Association of American Physicians, and I was also an Associate Professor of Research Medicine at the University of California. I started carrying around a small notebook, in which I wrote comments on my more unusual and instructive case records; later I used these records in writing various articles and a few books.

My first patient in the new office

I still remember my first patient, a woman of forty, who complained of a misery in her "stomach." After much study, I decided it was a "functional" trouble, due partly to her overly sensitive nervous system, and partly to her frequent distresses, trying to live with a "difficult" husband. On examining her thoroughly I found no sign of organic disease, but I did not tell her that there was "nothing the matter with her," as some of my friends used to do. I told her I was satisfied that her distresses were due partly to her overly sensitive nervous system, and partly to her distress of having to live with a hot-tempered husband. She thanked me and left. Later she returned to tell me that I had been wrong. A surgeon, on seeing her, said she had a "chronic appendix." He removed it surgically, and she said she was well. I thanked her for "contributing to my education." But after a while she returned to tell me that her misery had come back unchanged, so she had gone to another surgeon whose hunch was that her trouble was in her stoneless gall-bladder, so he had removed that. Again I thanked her, and again we parted good friends.

In three months she returned once more to say that when the misery had returned she had consulted a urologist who diagnosed a movable right kidney and had sewed it in place. When his huge bill came, her husband went into such a rage that her old distress instantly came back, worse than it ever had been. This time the lady said she had at least learned her lesson: she had finally come to see that her troubles were due to her husband's violent tantrums. She thanked me for never having thought up any scheme for making money out of her. After that she was a good and devoted patient. Strangely, one day, forty-eight years later, I heard from her, and she said she still had her old abdominal discomforts.

When I was an intern, I learned that in many cases abdominal pain or bloating can be due purely to nervousness, or perhaps to some annoyance in the home, office or factory. Also I learned to recognize "constitutional inadequates," people who had a life-long tendency to be getting one "misery" or bearable illness after another from youth to old age.

One of these unfortunate people, a young man of twenty or so, came to me first in 1912. I sensed then that with his many discomforts, he had been born "constitutionally inadequate." When I learned that his sister had had a spell of psychosis, I suspected that a mildly psychotic gene in him might be causing his tendency to suffer constantly from mild illnesses.

I lost track of him in 1926 when I left for Rochester, but in 1976, when he heard that I had returned to San Francisco, he twice called me on the telephone, and we had long chats. He told me that for all of his life he has had repeated ailments, mild enough so that he was able to work steadily in an office and earn a living. He is now retired. He never married.

Another constitutionally inadequate person, a pleasant but very sickly woman, I heard from the other day. She is still living in a general hospital with mild repeated illnesses. She came to me first in 1930 when she was twenty-five. When I and my associates in the Mayo Clinic studied her thoroughly — and found no sign of disease in her spine to explain her repeated spells of back-ache — we warned her not to have an operation on her spine. However, on her return home, an optimistic surgeon operated on her back, but succeeded only in making her a chronic hospital inmate. During the years since 1930, I have heard of only one interval when that poor woman was able to work (as a maid). Now, after forty-seven years, she tells me she still is miserable and living in a hospital.

The great Charles Darwin was constitutionally inadequate for most of his life. In his case the trouble was due apparently to his inheritance of nervous ill health from both his grandfather and his grandmother. His eccentric grandfather, Erasmus Darwin, had a depressed son who committed suicide, and Darwin's grandmother had a close relative who died "practically insane." Charles Darwin had a kindly brother who could never work, and so lived alone all his days. Charles Darwin had three depressions; four of his sons were depressed, and another son was feeble-minded. Charles was frail, and could work only three hours a day. In his last five years of life he was better, perhaps because his nerves were less sensitive. At seventy-three he died of a heart attack. His nerves were so sensitive that if he had guests for supper, he would lie awake most of the night and vomit during much of the next day.

The most remarkable abdominal pain I ever saw kept coming at weekly intervals, for years, to torment a good-looking young woman who did not seem very nervous. She lived in a nice home with her pleasant divorced mother. I went and visited them briefly in their home, and they seemed to be getting along together all right. What the young woman had were spells in which her anterior abdominal wall would become board-like, and with that there would come labor-like pains in the abdomen. These pains were so severe that only morphine would relieve them.

Several other physicians and I studied her carefully and found no sign of any organic disease. As I remember, a surgeon explored her abdomen and found nothing wrong. After a few years of such suffering, her mother died and immediately the woman was well! Then an old physician in the patient's city told me he felt sure what had caused the trouble: the young woman got her pains when her mother confessed that the girl was the illegitimate daughter of one of America's most eminent writers. The mother had tried hard to talk the man into marrying her, but he would not do it. The woman later married an unloved man just to give the girl a "father," but the girl so hated the fellow that the mother soon divorced him.

My doctor friend was satisfied that the young woman's illness was probably her unconscious way of punishing the mother for not getting for her the famous family name of her real father. Certainly, the day the mother died the young woman was well. Later, I saw a picture of her father, and was much impressed by the fact that she was the very image of him.

After seeing hundreds of patients with a duodenal ulcer that flared up again and again whenever the person had some great problem or annoyance, I was forced to conclude that duodenal ulcer is primarily a nervous disease, produced by distressing emotion. I was the surer of this when during the years when many men attacked me verbally for some of my writings, which they thought were all wrong and stupid, I sometimes had severe hunger pain. But 25 yearly X-ray studies failed to show any sign of an ulcer in either my stomach or duodenum. I called the disease "pseudo-ulcer." Along the way I saw some other physicians who suffered from hunger pain without any X-ray sign of an ulcer. One medical professor was so anxious to prove that I was crazy when I found no duodenal ulcer in him to explain his hunger pain, that twice he had his stomach and duodenum explored surgically, but neither time could an ulcer be found.

A certain doctor with whom I worked had such severe hunger pain that he always kept a big bottle of milk in his office. Although X-rays indicated that there was no ulcer, my associate jeered at my diagnosis of "pseudo-ulcer." Not long after, he had a severe stroke and died. An autopsy performed on him revealed that there was neither an ulcer nor the scar of an ulcer!

During the years when some physicians wrote letters jeering at me for "my stupidities," I rarely became upset nervously, but apparently the letters did produce some nervous tension, because the day I outlived nearly all of my severe critics, I had no more hunger pain!

Then I saw a young man with one of the worst ulcer pains I ever heard of. Every time he came to me for help, and I asked him what had brought on the spell of pain, he said the same thing, "I had a wordy fight with my father. He wants me to learn to run his huge business, and I won't have it." Then the young fellow disappeared for three years. When he came back from a strenuous life in the South Seas during the

American-Japanese war, he assured me that in spite of living on often poorly prepared "Army grub," he had never had a single spell of hunger pain! When I asked him why he had had no pain, he said, "Because my father could not get at me." His case and some others like his showed me that a special soft diet is not always necessary for the cure of an ulcer in the duodenum.

One day, many years ago, at a meeting of the American Medical Association, a big crowd of doctors listened to two internists who said that duodenal ulcers could be cured with bed rest and a diet. Then two surgeons got up and said that gastrointestinal ulcers could best be treated with an operation. I could sense that the doctors in the audience still had their doubts. Then the chairman called on me to start the discussion, and as I walked up to the platform with my knees shaking, wondering what to say, I thought of a helpful story. I told that crowd that the discussion made me think of a time when the Lord sent down on earth Saints Peter and Paul to see what was going on, and to report their findings. When lunch-time came they went into a restaurant. After lunch, the waiter brought them the dice-box so they could see who should pay the bill. Peter took the box, shook it, mumbled a few words, rolled out five sixes, and said, "All right, Paul, you can pay." But Paul shook the box, mumbled some words and rolled out five sevens! And Peter said, "Now Paul, no miracles between friends." With that, the doctors roared with laughter and understanding.

A tailor who I once treated for ulcers taught me to never again order the then standard Sippy treatment, consisting of a diet and a month in bed. When he was discharged from the hospital, he seemed to have been cured. But months later, when I had not heard from him, I went to see him. I learned that on returning to his shop such a disaster had befallen him that his ulcer had come raging back, worse than it had ever been. While he had been away, the man he had left in charge of the shop had decamped with the valuable list of his customers, all of his bolts of cloth, and worst of all, his wife! I felt so sorry for this poor fellow that I wished that I could give him a thousand dollars. But at that time, I too was almost broke. I never again used the Sippy treatment.

How remarkable that Plato, in the 5th Century B.C., warned

physicians not to try to cure the body without at the same time helping the soul. Also remarkable was the story by the great Michel de Montaigne, of a man who, several days after having given a dinner at his home, "bragged in jest (for no such thing had occurred), that the guests had partaken of a baked cat — at which a young gentlewoman, who had been at the feast, took such a horror, with violent vomiting and fever, that there was no possible way to save her!"

In 1917, I was asked by the United States Army to examine a number of young draft evaders to see if they were unfit for military service. In those days few physicians expected to find high blood pressure in young people, and so I was surprised to find in these young men that many had an abnormally high blood pressure. On learning that for years the doctors in the Student Health Service of the University of California had been recording the blood pressures of the entering freshmen, I obtained permission to analyze 15,000 of these measurements. In order to learn something about the pressures in children, I taught some of the physical education teachers in the San Francisco schools to make the necessary measurements, and they soon supplied me with hundreds of data. From all these figures I learned that high blood pressure commonly begins in children and young adults. In the years that followed, I published six papers containing what, so far as I could ever learn, were the first reliable standards of blood pressure, based on records of persons chosen pretty much at random, and not of persons chosen because their pressures had been found to lie within limits previously assumed to be normal by life insurance medical examiners.

As I tried to analyze my mass of records of blood pressures, I saw that I needed some knowledge of statistical practices. Accordingly, I bought the four best books then available on the subject, and absorbed their contents. I also went to Baltimore to talk over my problems with Dr. Raymond Pearl, the medical statistician. He was delighted to find that "at last a clinician was getting interested in statistical methods."

It was fortunate for me that, so early in my medical career, I learned something which I am sorry to say, is not always remembered today; this is that *abdominal pain* is often produced by some disturbance (emotional or physical) *up in the brain.* When I was an intern I learned to recognize the very painful "gastric crises" of late nervous syphilis, but it was many years before I came to see how commonly somewhat similar crises, often with retching, are due to migraine, epilepsy, psychoses, or hysteria. After 1955 I wrote several papers on this type of pain.

Many a time when my students just could not believe that a pain in a patient's abdomen could be due to something wrong in his brain, I used to tell them of the fine old doctor I saw once with pain in the pit of his stomach, so severe that the most probable diagnosis was a cancer of the pancreas. Then he died, and at autopsy his abdominal organs were found to be perfectly normal. He had died of a tumor in his brain.

A young woman who taught me much about abdominal pain coming from the brain was a lovely person of poor nervous heredity who, until she was 30, was an efficient office manager. Then a man who made his living by cheating women "borrowed" all of her savings, obstensibly to go and get a divorce and come back to marry her. He took her money, and she never saw him again. She developed a constant and very distressing pain in her right side — a pain which was not relieved by either an appendectomy or later the cutting of all the sensory nerves which leave the abdominal cavity. Eventually, she went into a depression and committed suicide. Her abdominal pain evidently had come out of her brain.

A nice-looking woman of 35, a gifted and clever but poorly adjusted business woman, could never be taught to keep living sensibly enough so as to maintain good mental and physical health. She could be charming, but she had little self-discipline, and little sense when it came to leading a well-ordered life.

The important point — so typical of such people — was that everytime I thought I had gotten her "on her feet," she would come tumbling down again. For years urologists had treated her for a pain that was supposed to be in her right kidney, but which, actually, was coming out of her stormy brain. Several times she had a chance to marry advantageously, but each time, at the last minute, she backed out because she felt she was entering a trap. Perhaps she knew in her heart that she was too independent, undisciplined, and self-centered ever to make a good wife for any man.

Another patient was the wife of a Nevada miner who one day struck a big vein of silver ore, so rich that it quickly made him wealthy. Soon he was being invited to the homes of well-to-do mining friends. However, he saw that his wife, whom years before he had picked up in a "House" in Reno, was in need of culture. So he paid a decayed gentlewoman — an old patient of mine in San Francisco — to "make a lady" of her. One noon, some weeks later, as the two women were having luncheon in the Court of the Palace Hotel in San Francisco, the miner's wife suddenly pointed to a large, bediamonded woman at a nearby table, and said, "Well, for crying out loud; if that ain't Carson City Lil; why, I once worked in her House; I wonder what the goddamned old bitch is doing here. Oh; excuse me for pointing!" Obviously, the pupil's manners were well on the way to improvement!

Around 1917 everyone who consulted a physician, even for an ingrowing toenail, was likely to be told, "Go and get all of your devitalized teeth extracted." Because it seemed to me that this was a fad from which we physicians should be recovering, I asked some 200 people who had each had several perfectly serviceable teeth removed, what they had gotten out of their sacrifice. And soon I found that few had gotten anything except a dentist's bill. Hence in 1919, I wrote a "Protest against the reckless extraction of Teeth." I think this paper eventually did some good.

I never liked the consultations of the old type, in which I would meet the family physician, listen to what he had to say, examine the patient, and then retire to a room to tell the doctor what I thought. If only because the patient was paying me, I felt he had a right to receive my honest opinion. In the old days most doctors thought that medical etiquette demanded that the consultant's main duty was to back up their diagnosis, and perhaps save them from criticism when they had made a bad mistake.

Because I could not bring myself to do this sort of thing, I never got a consultant practice in San Francisco. When I disagreed openly with a certain type of doctor, that was the last time he ever called me in. When

I asked a few old-time professional consultants how they had managed for 30 or 40 years to keep their practice, they admitted that they had always protected the doctors who had called them in.

Occasionally I found a physician whose honesty I greatly admired. After I had examined his patient he would say to me, "Go ahead and talk to the family right here; if I have been mistaken, so be it. I called you in because you know more about this type of illness than I do, and I want your help and guidance."

Incidentally, I have always loved the story a dear old doctor from Georgia told me about a consultation he once took part in. He told of an ailing old "Colonel" in Georgia who had agreed to accept a consultation with a physician from John Hopkins University. Shortly before the great professor arrived, the testy old patient called his butler and said, "Look, George; you know how these consultations go: the professor will come in and poke me here and there; then he and old Doc will go into my den for a drink. They'll talk over their golf scores; then they'll figure out what I am to be told, and then the professor will come and tell me a cheerful yarn. But I am not going to pay $1,000 for that. While they are in the den, you stand around and keep your ears open, and when they are gone you come and tell me exactly what they said."

So later, George came, and the Colonel started asking about the condition of his heart and his other organs. All went well until it came to the question of his kidneys, about which George was vague. As he said, "They just argued and argued about your kidneys." "But what," said the Colonel, "did they finally say was wrong with my kidneys?" "They didn t say, sir; they said the autopsy would show what's the matter with your kidneys!"

One thing I learned was that when I called a consultant I must choose a man, not because he would send me back a patient in return, but because he was the sort of able and honorable man I would choose to take care of my mother, my wife, or my child. There are several reasons for a young doctor's being honest in this matter. Let us say that when he has to refer a patient for an operation, he calls an incompetent surgeon, just because the man will send a "case" back to him, or will split his fee with him; some of the lay people and physicians in the town will soon know what he is doing, and their unpleasant remarks will do him harm.

When he refers a woman for an operation, she will ask her lay friends and a doctor or two about the "surgeon." If she hears good reports of the man, she will go to him with confidence; and then, if she is well treated, and gets a good result, she will be grateful to the internist who sent her. But if everywhere the woman asks, she hears, "I never heard of him," or "He's not much of a surgeon," she will be angry, and will have no more to do with the young man who made the referral.

Also, if the young physician wants to become one of the leading internists in his city, he had better start right off referring his patients only to the best surgeons, orthopedists, obstetricians, gynecologists, and other specialists in the town.

Early in my medical life I learned that commonly, if one goes ahead and does something that needs to be done, no one objects; but if one asks permission, and is refused, then the opposition is likely to become adamant. One day in came two nuns, the younger one — the patient — suffering from severe menstrual difficulties. After taking the history, I asked the older nun if it would be permissible for me to make a pelvic examination. She said she did not know, but would ask the Reverend Mother.

In a few days the Mother Superior telephoned that she was putting the question up to the local Archbishop. Later, when the Archbishop refused to decide the matter, the question was referred to the head of the Order in New York, and eventually, the Superior there wrote that the answer was, "No."

I then asked the Superior in New York if the examination might be made by a woman physician, and finally permission for this was granted. Ever since then, whenever a nun has come into my office for an examination, my nurse has had her undress and get up on the table like everyone else. And in 40 years, there was never one question or protest about it!

Often I was impressed by the fact that certain physicians have enough strength of character, or vividness of personality, or "magic" power to enable them to cope with "difficult," eccentric, or mildly psychotic people — especially hysterical women.

One day, while I was lunching with a colleague, a big handsome man came by. I glanced at his large, magnetic black eyes and said to my friend, "What a wonderful quack that man could be." And my friend said, "What an intuition you have: a while ago that man discovered that he has a remarkable ability to cure nervous women by the 'laying on of hands,' and so that is now his occupation."

Years ago I knew a surgeon who had this same remarkable ability to influence women. He had that "look" in his eyes, and he could quickly give a woman the impression that he had fallen for her in a big way. Because he was born overly shy, he compensated for this by being terribly profane with practically everyone. But for some reason, profanity coming from him did not offend anyone; in spite of it, his woman patients adored him.

One day he was asked to see the wife of a prominent Anglican bishop. She had gotten a fine room in the plushiest of the local hospitals, and she loved it there so much that she wouldn't get up and go home. The family doctor became worried because he just couldn't talk the woman into going back to her dull husband in his dreary "palace." So the doctor asked the surgeon to come and see what he could do. The story, as it was told to me by the woman's nurse, was that the surgeon came, looked over the record, quickly examined the old lady's heart, and then, for a few minutes, in his subtlest and most charming way, acted as if he had fallen in love with her.

Then, with the merriest twinkle in his eyes, he said, "Look; you goddamned old bitch, you don't need that bed any more than I do. You're not sick; you are just bored stiff with that prosaic old bishop of yours. So, come on now! Get up out of there, put on your clothes, and go home!"

She did exactly as she was told, and then, for the rest of her days, went around town telling everyone how she loved the surgeon for his "cute ways."

In a similar vein, I once treated a young girl who for two years had remained on a couch, with her widowed mother a slave to her. Seeing that the girl had no interest in getting well, I told her to go on home; I wasn't interested either, and had no time to waste on her. But I went ahead for a few minutes to paint a word picture of what her future was to be — without beaux, without a husband or a home of her own — just a dull, stupid life on a couch. Worse yet, when her old mother died, she (the girl) would be "buried alive" — alone in an apartment. Then I painted a picture of how much more fun she could have if she would get up and go back to school and college, and to a normal social life of dances and week-end parties.

After crying a while, she begged me to help her. Then she got up from her couch; she started eating, and she eventually went to college. Fattened up, she was a pretty girl. As she said, several doctors had failed to help her because she needed to be shaken out of her complacency. What startled her was to find a doctor who would have nothing to do with her unless she showed some desire to get well. Actually one of the biggest lessons I had to learn after I started practice is that one cannot cure anyone against his will. For several reasons many people need their disease; they use it to control or punish someone, or to get out of some unpleasant duty.

I always hate to see any sign of arrogance in a physician. I have known many a doctor who was so touchy that no patient was ever allowed to question what he had said. Naturally, this refusal to listen to a patient's objection must have led to many serious mistakes in diagnosis. I remember an occasion when I was asked to see a woman who was on her way to the hospital for a surgical exploration of her abdomen. She said, "Doctor, I fear your colleagues did not get my history correct; they all got the impression that I have abdominal *pain,* but that is wrong; what I have are spells of *nausea* with a *headache,* and some *abdominal soreness."* When I took another and more detailed history, it became clear that what the woman had was a severe migraine, and hence she did not need an operation.

The most beautiful example of the sort of mistake a physician can make when he *tells* his patient right off what is wrong, was made by a doctor who believed that every woman should have many children. When he was consulted by a handsome, well-dressed woman of 40, and learned that she had no children, he bristled at her and said, "I know your type well. You spend most the morning dolling yourself up;

you play cards in the afternoon, and you live a stupid indoor existence. What you need is to get out of doors, and to get some excitement into your dull life." As the woman said to me later, "I did not bother to tell him that my husband is head of a gang of men who smuggle Scotch whisky across the Canadian border. Most nights I sit in the car with him, holding a sub-machine gun across my knees, watching out for highjackers!"

Sometimes in those busy days in San Francisco I used to feel that I had to criticize some of the things that we physicians were doing. I felt it was my duty to do this, and that if I did not speak up, at some later date I would be ashamed of the fact that I had remained silent. As Abraham Lincoln said, "To sin by silence when they should protest makes cowards of men." Sometimes it is "base to sit dumb."

On several occasions — on principle — I stood up just to be counted as one of those few physicians in my state who was not fighting the much-needed Workmen's Compensation laws.

The man who runs athwart the current of his time is bound to gain some unpopularity, and most of us hate to be unpopular; we would much prefer to be known for our genial good nature. But we must remember that only the man who never does anything outstanding can go through this life without running into opposition, dislike, and bitter criticism.

We have to remember that "A turtle can never get anywhere unless he sticks his neck out!" I would have much liked to be always popular, but I did not care to buy my popularity at the price of remaining silent when I felt that someone should speak out against unwise, purely commercial, or heartless types of medical practice.

After 1925, I kept wishing I could find some institution that would give me a laboratory and just enough money for me and my family to live on. Each month I kept watching the medical journals, looking for some place to which I might go — but I never heard of one.

And then, late in 1925, I had the good fortune to be invited to give a number of lectures in Salt Lake City and Pocatello. At the final banquet, my good angel saw to it that I was seated beside Dr. William Braasch, a member of the Board of Governors of the Mayo Clinic. When he learned from me that I was unhappy in San Francisco, and anxious to make any move that would give me more time for study, he went back and told Dr. Will Mayo, who promptly invited me to join the Staff of the Mayo Clinic. One glance at the letter that came, and I said to my secretary, "Goodby, I am going!"

One of the pleasantest memories I have of the days when I was leaving San Francisco is of the farewell luncheon that a number of my friends in the two medical schools gave me when I left. There were several very kind speeches made, but I particularly remember a few sentences out of the summing-up talk made by Walter Boardman, Professor of Medicine at Stanford. He said, "Walter, there are men who, if they had risen to prominence as fast as you have done in the last ten years, would have brought on themselves envy and jealousy, but you have not excited any such ill feelings, because we all know that what you have won has been gained, not at the expense of any one of us — your competitors for a consultant practice — but by the hardest sort of work in the laboratory, the library, and the clinic."

Because of these affectionate words, I left that luncheon with feelings of humility and warmth in my heart, and gladness because in this world what are most worthwhile are not money and honors, but the esteem, good will and affection of the men and women who know if one's work has been good and honest.

CHAPTER IX

1926-1950

On February 1st, 1926, my family and I arrived in Rochester, Minnesota, and I went to work in the Mayo Clinic. My first months were particularly happy because every day I was learning something at the several seminars and Staff meetings. I could so quickly and easily get answers to the many questions that were in my mind. Often all I had to do was to talk to a colleague who was an authority on the particular subject that was then interesting me. Sometimes, in one week, I would see so many people with the same rare disease that I could quickly become well acquainted with its clinical picture.

For instance, in 1926 there were so many patients with exophthalmic goiter walking about the streets of Rochester that even our observant laymen, on noticing the bulging eyes, the dark red skin, and perhaps the operative scar on the neck, could instantly make the diagnosis.

My good friend Dr. Alfred Kinsey once told me that when his little boy began to show signs of exophthalmic goiter, he had a hunch what was wrong, because he had watched a relative suffering from the disease. Because the local professor of pediatrics hooted at the idea of a small boy's ever having a toxic goiter (actually it *is* very rare in a child), Dr. and Mrs. Kinsey took the boy to Rochester. There, a small girl in the hotel promptly called out, "Hey! You with the poppy eyes! You'd better go have your goiter cut out!" She had made the correct diagnosis in an instant, when a teacher of pediatrics had failed! I remember when a newsboy made this diagnosis and astonished a much-traveled patient as he got off the train at Rochester. His examination at the Clinic

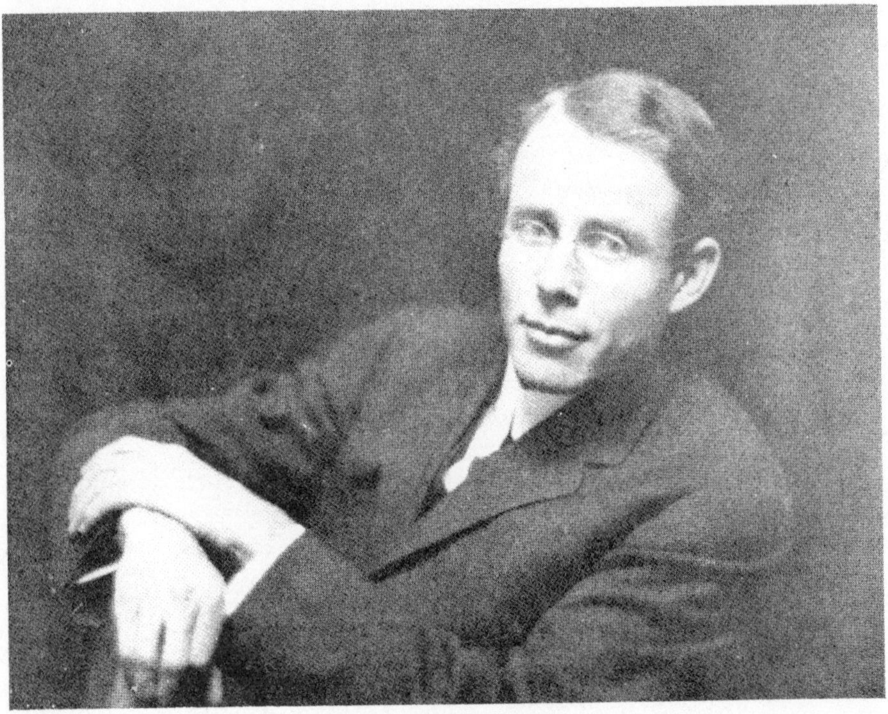

Me, in about 1920

showed that the newsboy was right.

My mornings were spent in my laboratory in the basement of St. Mary's hospital. My assistant and I worked so hard that in one year we had published over a dozen articles. Dr. Arnold Zimmerman and I made the first movies of the actively contracting stomach and bowel of an anesthetized rabbit, with the abdomen open under a bath of warm saline solution. These movies were shown over the next year or so at many major medical meetings.

With the assistance of George Little (our chief mechanic), I designed an X-ray motion picture machine, which, I am happy to report, performed admirably. This apparatus allowed me to record the passage of waves up and down the bowels of still conscious animals.

My life at Mayo's was always interesting, if only because "the world and his wife" was constantly streaming through Rochester. Many delightful people came, not only from all over America, but from the four corners of the globe as well.

One day my wife and I had in our home for luncheon a Chinese, two Australians, two Canadians, a South African, a South American, and two physicians from this country. In all, Harriet and I entertained over 600 persons. And I was pleased that our children could meet many famous people, and to find that usually the greater the man, the more approachable he is, and the more at home one almost immediately feels with him. I remember the evening when my old friend Paul DeKruif was in our home, and our daughter Bernice, then 14, whispered, "Daddy, do you think he would come down to the High School and talk to our journalism class?" I said, "Go ask him." And I remember his booming answer, "But, dear, what will I talk about?" I remember also, a few minutes later, the charming picture of the great big man and the young girl walking down the street together, hand in hand — having a grand chat!

One evening my wife and I learned something about entertaining the "great." The day before Christmas I was chatting with one of the most distinguished generals in the U.S. Army Medical Corps — a big handsome man with many rows of service ribbons on his coat. Becase of his eminence, I felt sure he would be spending Christmas Eve in one of our "great houses;" but I asked anyway, and learned that everyone had thought that someone else was taking care of him, and hence no one was. Accordingly, I invited him to our home, and he gladly accepted. That bitter cold evening my wife and I put together two card tables by the fireplace; we had a happy dinner there with much good conversation, and then the general came out into the kitchen with us and helped me wipe the dishes, as my wife washed them.

Later we received the sweetest letter from this much-traveled man, saying that many a time he had dined in state, he had dined with kings; but never had he enjoyed a dinner more than the one that was served on card tables by a crackling fire.

Every morning I was in my office at eight. Especially on Mondays, over 1,000 new patients might come streaming into the Clinic buildings. They would be registered and each assigned to one of the several "Diagnostic Sections." In most of these Sections, the doctors tended to specialize, as in heart disease, or diabetes, or allergy, or diseases of the lungs, or stomach, or bowels. Thus, I, in a "stomach section," saw an occasional patient with a bad heart or bad lungs. But in most cases, if the problem was at all puzzling, I would quickly call a heart or a lung consultant and turn the patient over to him. One of the wonderful features about practice in the Mayo Clinic is the ease and quickness with which a doctor can call a consultant; also the honesty and the openness with which the consultations are held — always in the presence of the patient.

After being registered, a patient who (unless he is bedfast) stays in a hotel or a boarding-house, is assigned to a Fellow — a young physician who, after finishing his internship and residency, has come to the Clinic to work for 3 years as a graduate student of the University of Minnesota. This Fellow takes the first history and makes a physical examination. Then one of the men of the "Permanent Staff" consults, and perhaps OK's the orders made for laboratory and X-ray work. When this work is done and he sees the patient again, he may re-take the history and re-axamine the patient, and perhaps with this he can make the diagnosis. If not, he orders more examinations or tests. Later he may consult with someone, or he may arrange for an operation or some special treatment, or he may dismiss the person. Then, in many a case, he dictates a report to the patient's home physician.

Each patient gets one bill. Close to a third of the patients, because of their financial problems, are given all the time they need to pay their bill. No one has ever been sued for payment, and no one has ever been turned away because his purse was empty.

One thing I have always loved and admired about the Mayo Clinic practice is that there has never been any buncombe in it — no carrying-out of long treatments that are not needed; operating on people who do not need an operation, and no ordering of tests just to run up a big bill. Actually, there were times when Dr. Will and Dr. Charlie called the Staff together, and begged us to try to hold down the size of the bill — particularly for people who had little money. One day Dr. Will was distressed when he found that a poor young tenant farmer, who had come in with a mangled hand, had had three expensive transfusions of blood. As Dr. Will said, a husky young chap like him could almost certainly have recovered without the help of the blood. Some salt solution in his veins would have worked about as well.

Another time, Dr. Will called a meeting to discuss the foolishness and unkindness of ordering great numbers of tests which, with a little thought, could have been "done without." Our Fellows used often to order dozens of tests without much thinking — perhaps because in their University hospitals they had been allowed to do this, or even taught to do it. As Dr. Will said, it is not honest to take money for unneeded tests. Eventually, a regulation had to be passed to the effect that tests asked for by a Fellow could not be made until each order had been approved by a consultant.

Naturally, for an ardent student of disease like me, it was wonderful to see so many patients, and particularly those many who came because their trouble was so rare and puzzling that their home doctors could not guess what it was. Each day was full of diagnostic challenges which I greatly enjoyed. I was taking particular pleasure in helping patients who I found were ill only because of a great sorrow, or a great strain of some kind.

Typical was the story of the banker who had been traveling about the

United States consulting eminent physicians in an effort to find out what was causing the pain in his abdomen. After much study, one of my associates dismissed him with the statement that there was "nothing the matter with him." Naturally, the man was disappointed and outraged. Then, while strolling past a book store he saw my book in the window, *Nervousness, Indigestion and Pain.* Thinking he might learn from this how to make his own diagnosis, he went in and bought a copy.

Later he came to my office and told my secretary he just had to see me and tell me that as soon as he had read the first chapter, a great light had dawned on him. It had never occurred to him before that his pain could be due to some distressing emotion, but as he looked through my book he saw that it could. Suddenly, the thought came to him that he never felt the pain when he was away from home — at a bankers' convention, on his ranch, or on his fishing preserve; and then he realized that the minute he went home and stuck the key into his door, he would get it.

I asked, "What is your wife like?" And he said, "She is a good woman, but she is always looking down her nose at me. She had a college education, and I didn't finish high school. She was born up on the hill, and I was born below the railroad tracks. So she tells me I am common. She does not like my English, or my table manners, or my friends. At home she won't let me kick off my shoes, and she won't let me smoke in the living-room. She won't let me bring my poker-playing cronies in the house. She always manages to keep me tense and uncomfortable."

"Well, you now know how to cure your stomach-ache; just keep away from home."

"That," he said, "is precisely what I am going to do. From now on, I am going to live alone on my ranch."

One of the patients I saw in 1926 found himself faced with such a strange problem that, in my mind's eye, I can still see the poor old fellow. He was a man of sixty who for most of his life had run a general store in a small town in North Dakota. When some indigestion began to bother him, he went to a doctor who had just bought an X-ray machine, and didn't yet know much about it. When the films of the man's stomach showed a big indentation, the doctor diagnosed an inoperable cancer.

When the man came to Rochester and showed me these films, I laughed and said "That isn't a cancer; that apparent deformity is produced by the pressure of your spine on your stomach." As the man continued to look sad and apathetic, I asked, "What is the matter? You should be registering joy and great mental relief!"

"Oh, Doctor," he said, "I don't know what I am going to do; I am in an awful fix. When the doctor said I would soon be gone, I gave the store to my son. All I saved out was some money for a trip to Rochester and a funeral! The townspeople were so kind and so wonderful to me; they all came down to the railroad station to say goodbye to me; and now they do not expect ever to see me again. I just can't go back! It would be such an awful anticlimax. I do not know where to go!"

One day I had another strange experience with an unusual patient, and learned something from her I had not known before. I learned that Saint Peter must make pelvic examinations on very proper maiden ladies whose main claim to the right to enter heaven is that they always kept their virginity. What happened was that a very wealthy and very proper old maid came up from South America for the removal of a large tumor of her womb. A few months after her return home, I was surprised to have her come in again. She said that she had returned just to get from me a certificate to the effect that the loss of her hymen had come about perfectly innocently during her several medical and surgical examinations. She had discovered her loss when, on her return to Lima, her prissy old Spanish doctor had checked her over and had been horrified to find that an extremely important little portal had become somewhat dilated. When I asked her what she was going to do with her certificate, she said that, of course, it was going with her in her coffin to be presented in due time to St. Peter. I had never before realized that the Saint or some deputy of his at the gates of Heaven must perform pelvic examinations on all would-be entrants who claim to be"virgo intacta!"

Although my quarter-century at the Clinic was the most fortunate and productive period of my life, I must admit that occasionally I ran into trouble with a few of my associates, and a few committees made up of men who doubted the wisdom or advisability of what I wanted to do. Often I must have appeared to them as an *enfant terrible.* Certainly I was not the quiet, retiring, and conforming man who is most likely to get along comfortably as a simple cog in a great machine. I was too full of ideas for doing something new.

I never wanted "to rock the boat," but sometimes I blundered into doing this if only because, when I arrived in Rochester, no one told me of all the many unwritten laws and "feelings of personal rights" around the place — "rights" that must be respected. Some of the men at times tried to block what I was doing, usually, I think, because they were not convinced that I was right in what I was reporting, or because they feared that what I wanted to do would injure the medical standing of the Clinic, or it would make enemies for the place.

I just could not get them to see that my coming did not constitute any threat to them. All I wanted was to be left alone to work, study and learn; I did not want anyone's job or anyone's patients. I did not want to be head of a department; I did not want even a hospital appointment. I guess my associates' trouble was that they just could not imagine how a man could have as little ambition as I claimed to have. I was full of a desire to work, but the work I wanted to do was in research, not in administration.

Everywhere I went in medical schools and clinics I found that a man who does not fit into a well-recognized groove in an organization is bound to run into trouble. As my old associate Dr. McVicar used to say, "Walter, for God's sake, either fish or cut bait. *You* want to do both!" One of my troubles arose from the fact that in my mornings I worked as a physiologist in my laboratory, and afternoons I worked as a consultant on the Clinic "Floor." Naturally, the physiologists said I was a clinician, and the clinicians said I was a physiologist!

Furthermore, a man will surely have trouble as I did if, when something urgently needs to be done, he does it without waiting until two or three committees have discussed it at length and decided to block it.

As I traveled about, hearing of the difficulties encountered by able men in many institutions, I thought often of what my great hero, Sir

Francis Galton, once wrote. He told how, in South Africa, the lions used to pick off and pull down just those oxen that were fearless enough and independent enough to *graze away from the herd.* In a land where the grass was deep and lions were numerous, practically all of the cattle, while grazing, felt comfortable only when gathered in a circle with their rumps together and their sharp horns facing outward.

But in every herd there were one or two oxen, brave enough or independent enough or perhaps foolish enough to graze off away by themselves. Naturally, in doing this, a steer ran a great risk, because a lion, sneaking up behind, could jump on his back and break his neck. Because independence with courage is apparently inherited, and because the lions destroyed most of the *brave animals* early in their life, there could never be many born into a herd.

Galton became much interested in these cattle with the independent-grazing habit because, while exploring in the desert, he used heavy carts pulled by perhaps ten pairs of oxen; and the biggest problem of the carters was to find two *"lead animals"* with enough courage to walk ahead, especially when the scent of lions was in the air. The average ox — like many an average man — *would never lead;* and the minute it became frightened, it would turn back and snarl up the team by trying to hide itself between the two lines of animals.

But here is the important point: early in their life in South Africa the Boers discovered that the only animals that could ever be trained to be leaders were just those rare brave ones that *would graze away from the herd.* Because of this, the Boers always watched for these particular cattle, and prized them highly.

I think of this story whenever in an organization I see men sneaking up behind the lead-ox type of man with plans to pull him down. Being attacked is the price many an able man must pay for being fearless, independent, progressive, willing to lead, and willing to graze away from the herd. Many men in this world will always refuse to accept responsibility — because they don't want to lead and they don't want to make decisions; they are too afraid of the criticism that would follow a mistake. A man who is "going to the top" must have guts enough to risk making many a mistake.

An adage that many a highly successful man must learn and get used to is that "When you want to beat a dog, any old stick will do." This saying has often occurred to me as I have watched an able man taking a verbal beating for having done a splendid piece of work. Take the life of Linnaeus — the great organizer of the science of botany. On one occasion jealous associates who wanted to pull him down and have him imprisoned, attacked him because he had shown that plants have two sexes! This discovery was regarded by the small men around him as so reprehensible that only Linnaeus' friendship with the king saved him from serious trouble.

Oliver Wendell Holmes once said that "doctors are the best-natured people in the world, except when they get to fighting each other."

I wish all committee men who now compel the research workers in their institution to stay in one narrow rut would remember that insulin was discovered by a country surgeon who got an idea and followed it up. Obviously, the drug should have been found by a physiologist — but it wasn't! Penicillin was found first by a bacteriologist. Years later it was isolated and purified by some chemists. Still later, it was made in bulk with the help of techniques borrowed from the brewers. The sulfa drugs were found by Gerhard Domagk — a pathologist.

Pasteur's life is the best illustration of what great gifts can come to the world when a man of genius strays from one field of endeavor to another. As we all know, Pasteur left his field of chemistry to found the sciences of bacteriology and immunology. With this work he changed the whole face of medicine. If he were in America today, the committee of his institution would quickly order him to go back into his chemical laboratory and stay there!

Often the only way I could learn something new about the functions of the digestive tract was to go out searching into other fields — like the fields of anatomy and physiology, and sometimes into the field of veterinary physiology.

Once, long ago when an old friend of mine — a professor of physiology — was commissioned to write a summary of that day's knowledge of the emptying of the stomach, he made no mention in his article of what was by far the best planned and best executed piece of work ever done on this subject. It was performed in my laboratory by a brilliant young roentgenologist, Dr. Cesare Gianturco, who used my X-ray movie machine. We used an ideal motion-picture technique in which the animal was wide awake, frisky, happy, and digesting a meal, and without the usual anesthesia, and surgically opened abdomen, or balloon in his stomach, or a tube running down his gullet. When I asked my friend, the professor, why he hadn't done Gianturco the courtesy of at least criticizing his work, he said (as I knew he would) that Gianturco and I were not full-time physiologists. We weren't full time "members of the union" so we had to be punished.

Once or twice, especially in my first years at the Clinic, when I ran into annoyances I thought of going back to San Francisco; but then I said to myself, "No; there is no bed of roses anywhere. In so many ways the Clinic is a wonderful place in whick to work, with every advantage, so why leave?" Perhaps also it is true, as Mark Twain used to say, that a certain number of fleas are good for a dog! One thing I fortunately learned early in mylife is that when harassed by someone, I must never waste any energy getting angry, or trying to strike back; *a man is never so poorly employed as when defending himself!*

Throughout all my years of writing, I kept having difficulties with committees, especially editorial committees. I had the worst times with young women who thought it their duty to rewrite almost every sentence in my articles and editorials. They always tried hard to make my work sound "more scientific" by putting in a lot of long Greek words — replacing my simple English words.

What has bothered me much about many editors has been their insistence always that I "pussyfoot." Many an article of mine has come back to me from some editorial office with every strong sentence blue-pencilled, and every statement that did not follow the "party line" ripped out. Time and again I have had to tell the editor or his assistant that if I had always consented to the emasculation of my prose, with the deletion of every strong sentence that someone feared would cause comment or make for me an enemy, my writing would never have had any influence on American medicine.

Once when I much wanted to impress physicians with the need for their more quickly diagnosing cancer of the stomach, I decided that the best way in which to stir up their interest would be to show them what a disgracefully poor job of diagnosing gastric cancer had been done *on themselves* by the last 41 physicians seen at the Clinic with the disease. In 20 of these cases the doctors had waited an average of 12 months before doing anything about their symptoms. One eminent stomach specialist suffered a year with pain typical of gastric cancer before he came to see me and was X-rayed. Another physician suffered two and one-half years before getting a diagnosis! A physician who lost 40 pounds waited a year before he got examined!

One of the editors who saw my manuscript demanded that I delete everything that would suggest I was criticizing the diagnostic ability of the doctors. Obviously, this would have left the article pointless. Not only would the Cheshire cat have disappeared; even its grin would have been wiped out; so I published the paper as it was.

The most awful "storm" of all was kicked up by a paper of mine on *abdominal ticklishness in women!* In 1913, when every afternoon I had to palpate the stomachs of people standing back of my X-ray screen, I found only a rare woman with an abdomen as ticklish as that of a boy. Becoming curious about this, for years I kept making notes about every decidedly ticklish woman whom I found. Finally, when I wrote a paper about these odd women, and mentioned the fact that in loveplay it would be somewhat of a handicap for a woman to have a very ticklish abdomen, my medical friends went into such paroxysms of horror that I yielded to their entreaties, and left the paper in my files, where it still is! How prissy we doctors can sometimes be! I can remember when a medical editor did not want me to mention sex or homosexuality in his august columns!

Very remarkable also was the "fit" many of my friends had when I turned in the manuscript of a paper I had written on those many persons who are ill because they feel "caught in a trap." My friends were so distressed over this paper that I gave in and put it away. When, a few years ago I took it out and published it, the response from the medical profession warmed my heart. Teachers of medicine all over the country kept writing in to ask for reprints, and to say how much they loved that paper, which "much needed to be written."

Here are a few items from it to show how harmless it was. One day I saw a girl who, because of her failure to eat, had gone down to skin and bones. I learned that her illness had begun when her half-crazy, sex-hating mother in Los Angeles had insisted that the girl give up her good job in Salt Lake City, dismiss her fiance, and come home. The mother had taken to her bed with the unwarranted conviction that she was dying, and she insisted that the daughter stay and take care of her until the end came.

What with the girl's worry about her beau, and her dull stupid life in a darkened room where her mother read the Bible all day, the girl's nerves had gone to pieces. I immediately got her father to promise to set her free, and to let her go back to her fiance and her job. When he agreed to do this, the girl started eating and gaining weight. During the next few years she kept writing to me to thank me, to say she was well, and happily married.

Some patients were trapped by feelings of guilt or great responsibility. I will never forget one of the saddest women I ever saw. She was desperately unhappy. Eventually she confessed to me that her great sorrow and her illness came when, on waking one night, and hearing someone in the kitchen, she went there to investigate, and found her husband taking a big drink of whiskey.

Because she was a devoted member of the Women's Christian Temperance Union, she felt so outraged that she gave him a savage scolding. He said nothing and just went back to bed. In the morning she found him dead. The family doctor, when questioned, asked, "Didn't your husband tell you that he had been suffering greatly with the anginal pain produced by a diseased heart? Didn't he tell you that the medicine that often gave him some relief was whiskey?" "No," said the wife, "he never told me a word about that." For long after that she suffered with her great feeling of guilt — because her last words with her husband had expressed so much wrath and scorn. She felt that she would be cured if she could only get five minutes with him to apologize abjectly for what she had said.

Fortunately for me, in my many years at Mayo's, the Editors-in-Chief — from Mrs. Maud Mellish, to Richard Hewitt, to Lloyd Potter, and to my good buddy James Eckman — always came to my rescue; they chased away the young ladies with the blue pencil, and along the way, they became my dear friends.

When I began working in the "stomach section" of the Mayo Clinic in 1926, I found that every man in the department had already been assigned some organ or disease as his field for special study. Accordingly, I had to ask, "What is there left for me?" And my associates said, "The digestive neuroses. You can have them all. We don't want them. We don't like 'neuros.' It takes too long to make anything out of their stories."

The subject of neuroses suited me perfectly. Thus it came about that for the next 25 years I studied the problems of thousands of patients with stomach-aches for which no abdominal cause had been found. Soon I showed that usually in these cases the diagnosis can be made only with the help of a carefully-taken and well-interpreted history.

Naturally, as the years passed, and I saw all these people with neuroses, migraine; "nervous breakdowns," little strokes, hysteria, mild and seizureless forms of epilepsy, and mild psychoses, my major interests changed, and soon I found myself spending most of my time trying to help people, not with ulcers or cancers, but with nervousness, worry, and fear. Before long I was writing books on gastrointestinal neuroses.

Along the way, seeking help, I went into the library and read widely on mental and nervous troubles. I particularly enjoyed the books and articles written by the older psychiatrists — men of great wisdom, like S. Weir Mitchell of Philadelphia, T. A. Ross, the great research psychiatrist of England, Austen Riggs, Abraham Myerson, Stanley Cobb, Hervey Cleckly, and others. They became my teachers and my heroes.

I was spending much of my time teaching my students to watch out for the thousands of persons who came complaining of aches and pains, but who really should have been telling stories of great sorrow, unhappiness, overwork with fatigue and insomnia, worry, strain, feelings of guilt, or feelings of distress over an inability to make an important decision.

A married woman of 45 came 1,000 miles just (she said) to have her gallbladder removed. She was much annoyed when I did not immediately send her into a hospital for the operation, and much more annoyed when I told her that not only were her symptoms those of a neurosis, but the X-ray study had shown her gallbladder to be normal. For ten days I verbally wrestled with that woman; I, asking her what had gone wrong in her life, and she saying, "Go on and get my gallbladder out." As I pointed out to my assistant on the first day, there must have been something wrong in the woman's sexual life because she had asked me if, with her examination, she would get a Wasserman test for syphilis.

On the tenth day she gave in and told me that her troubles had started when a woman had come to her door to say that her (my patient's) husband was a bigamist and her children were illegitimate because the man had never bothered to get a divorce before marrying again. This woman then blackmailed my patient into giving her $5,000 — to keep her mouth shut. The husband admitted his guilt, but said, "Pay no attention to Alice; she always was a bluffer!"

Sometimes I got to thinking that I was pretty good in suspecting the presence of such unhappy stories, and then getting the patient to confess; but sometimes I would run into a case in which I found that I had failed badly.

For instance: I failed to help a stout, fortyish, prosaic-looking farmer's widow whom I certainly never suspected of having any love problem. Because she complained of abdominal pain, I had to check her carefully to rule out a cancer. Twice she came, and twice I sent her home with the admission that I did not know what was wrong. Then I received a letter from her telling me what had been wrong. She had been too ashamed to tell me that her trouble was that ever since her husband's death she had been constantly distressed by her great hunger for sex. She had hoped that I would ask her about the subject because then she would have had the courage to ask me if there wasn't some sort of an operation that would give her peace and relief. "Each time you failed me," she wrote, "and so I wasted my money."

A frequent trouble I had with many of my nervous patients was that it was hard to help them when I could see them only occasionally. I had to tell them that most of the time by themselves they would have to fight their fears, worries, and feelings of illness. As Shakespeare said, "The patient must minister to himself."

Some of my patients amused me much, and many of them pleased me with their signs of great gratitude. Two of my most grateful patients were notorious gangsters who, strange to say, I came to like. One of them, a well-known citizen of Chicago, was so very grateful for the removal of a painful gallstone that he kept begging me to commit some crime so that through his friends he could quickly and easily "get me off!"

The other man kept asking if there wasn't someone whom I would like to have "bumped off." He assured me this would be done quickly and without any expense to me! All I was ever able to get him to do for me was to have a parking ticket "fixed!"

In my years at the Mayo Clinic I never came to feel that "I belonged." When talking to an audience about some Clinic practice, I unconsciously would say, *"they"* do so and so, and not *"we."* Dr. Will Mayo sensed this, and with his usual homely wisdom and kindliness he tried to comfort me.

He said, "Don't worry, Alvarez; a rat has to live in a strange garret for a good many years before he is accepted as one of the gang!"

Around 1930 I had the pleasure of having as an assistant a brilliant young woman, Dr. Frances Vanzant of Houston. Together we wrote six research papers, mainly on the gastric juice. One paper was on the technique of diagnosing with a computer. In the 1930's I spent much time studying food allergy, also the — to me — always fascinating syndrome of the "little strokes." Those strokelets, rarely causing any paralysis, but often some mental deterioration, are exceedingly common in the later years of many persons, and they have most to do with the aging of many of us.

Although I did not begin to lecture about these little strokes until the early 1930's, I came to know them well in the years from 1901 to 1911, as I watched a series of them slowly pull down and kill the brilliant college president who, in 1907, became my father-in-law.

Later I discovered that Osler had known the syndrome well, and had written briefly about those people "who take longer to die than they did to grow up." In the years following 1930 I wrote a number of papers describing the several groups of symptoms commonly produced by these little strokes. I am happy to say that general practitioners and lay people all over the world quickly accepted this work. Many doctors knew the disease well, if only because they had seen it develop in members of their own families.

When I first described — at a medical convention — the slow, steplike mental death of some of the people who keep having little strokes, a number of fine old family doctors came up to the platform and said, "How could we have been so stupid as not to recognize the nature of this very common disease? Why, right now in our town, we must have dozens of patients petering out in that way — dying at the top like an old tree."

My old friend Dr. James Kernohan, one of the most experienced brain pathologists in the world, often told me that the commonest lesion he kept finding in brains (removed at autopsies) had been a series of little black spots which represent plugged-up arteries (little strokes).

In October, 1931, Harriet and I left for a trip to Europe. We travelled through Ireland, France, Spain, Germany, Switzerland, Austria, and finally, England. It was there that I had such delightful visits with several professors. One night we had dinner at "High Table" with the Dons at Kings College, Cambridge. We gathered together in a large room where each of us donned a cap and gown. We then filed into the dining hall, and stood around the "High Table" (which is called so because the student dining area is situated about ten feet below where we sat), while a student scuttled rapidly through the long grace in Latin. We sat down, enjoying the stimulating company of the many renowned scholars who sat with us.

Later, in London, my wife and I had an interesting dinner with Dr. and Mrs. Ryle. He was a fine idealistic man — one of England's best internists and stomach specialists. He had his office on Wimpole Street, which is much like Harley Street — a row of ancient residences, each full of the offices of specialists. What surprised me was that about

8:30 P.M., after the last patient had left, a table was brought into the *waiting room* which was then converted into the *dining room!* Imagine such a thing happening in a big city in the United States!

While I was visiting with one of my good friends, a professor of comparative anatomy at Oxford, he told me that in his work he dissected animals that had died in the London Zoo. One day he got a message saying a lioness had died, and if he wanted the entrails, he should come and get them. So he picked up his specially-built suitcase, with its metal lining that could be screwed down until it was watertight, and left for the City.

Before returning home he checked the suitcase and took the train for home. On arriving, he ran up to his laboratory to leave the material in the refrigerator. When he opened the suitcase he was astonished to find that the baggage man had given him a case that looked like his, but wasn't; it contained the robes and regalia of a Grand Master of the Masons!

For several days my friend kept in touch with the baggage man, and watched the papers for a "personal," but the grand master never peeped; he was not going to go on trial in Old Bailey as a trunk murderer — not he! My friend said he would have given good money to have seen the face of the Grand Master as he opened that suitcase!

On our way through Ireland, just for fun, I climbed up onto the top of Blarney Castle, and with a man sitting on my legs, I leaned far out backward and kissed Blarney Stone.

In Vienna I sat at luncheon with Franz Lehar, the composer of "The Merry Widow." He was then a striking-looking man with a head of thick gray hair. I was surprised to see how quiet he was and how little inclined to chat. My greatest joy in Vienna was to go to a Hungarian restaurant where the Gypsy music was delightful.

After returning from Europe I went down to Mexico to speak at a meeting of the Mexican Medical Association. The meeting was held in what was said to be the oldest university building in the New World. The next day a friend drove me over to Patzcuaro, perhaps the most deeply religious town in a deeply religious land.

There I had a touching experience. I was strolling through the market place; it was a "feast day" and on every side there were gaily decorated booths where little articles of native manufacture were offered for sale. Some of the booths were filled with the cheapest of toys; little carts made of baked clay, much like those that are found in Mesopotamia in the graves of little children who died 5,000 years ago.

Walking just ahead of me was a Mexican Indian, in his white cotton suit, his floppy straw hat, his colorful *serape* over his shoulder, and his straw sandals on his feet. Holding on to his left hand was the cutest little black-eyed girl about five years old. She kept saying in Spanish, "Papacito (dear little father) please won't you buy me one of those little clay carts: I want one so much," and each time the Indian would say so sadly, "Dear little darling of my heart, I can't buy one because I have 'ni un centavo' — not a cent of money."

On impulse, I reached up to the woman in the nearest booth; I gave her the needed 35 centavos, and got one of the little wagons. Then, walking up silently behind the child, I slipped the toy into her chubby little hand. She just grasped it without looking back to see whence it had come. The father also did not notice what had happened because at the moment he was looking in another direction. The two just walked silently up the street.

Later that afternoon I heard people saying that a miracle had taken place that day in the holy city of Patzcuaro; a little Indian girl had prayed to the Blessed Virgin of Guadalupe for a clay cart, and behold, her prayer had been granted, and she had found the toy in her hand!

Through all my years at Mayo's I helped scores of young men to get their training in internal medicine. I did this usually in an informal way: perhaps just by showing an assistant how I would go at the problem of studying a particular patient; what tests I would order, and particularly — how I would take a long *history,* and then interpret it.

Some few of the more earnest students would ask if they might be in the room when I checked upon the history, or when I told the patient what had been found and what I thought he should do to get well. The best Fellows always, when a patient with an interesting problem was dismissed, went to the man's history sheets to see what their Chief had found that they had not found, and what he had disregarded — after they had thought it important.

My main difficulty in teaching the Fellows was to convince them that in many cases a psychic factor was far more important than was the gallstone, or muscular nodule on the womb, or inguinal hernia that they had found.

I had the same trouble with patients. Many a highly nervous woman so ached and hurt all over that she could not believe that "it was all nerves." Her only reaction to my diagnosis was to say I had not made enough tests. She was sure more examinations would reveal some terrible disease, and so she left to go and find a doctor who would make more tests.

In trying to convince people that a neurosis can oftentimes hurt even more than a cancer does, I used to tell the true story of a farmer's wife and her daughter. The nice old mother of 65 had a big cancer in her stomach, but because she was an "insensitive person," she had no pain or indigestion. She said, "Don't bother with me, I'm not sick; it is my daughter here who is very ill." What was wrong with the daughter? On coming home from the town where she was teaching school, and hearing what had been found wrong with her adored mother, she had begun to vomit every meal. By the time I saw her, she was so worn out and dried out that I had to send her into a hospital for the intravenous injection of some fluid.

So there before me were two women: one with the worst possible disease of the stomach — and no symptoms; and the other with no disease in her abdomen but with very distressing symptoms. Cicero once said so truly that, "The sufferings of the mind are more severe than the pains of the body."

In hundreds of cases, no matter what localized disease I might find and remove from the body of a person born frail and "inadequate," I could not work a "cure." In this connection I will never forget the thin, sickly little minister who came to consult me because of general discomforts affecting his whole body. Significant was the fact that his "miseries" always hit him hardest Sunday night after the evening service in his little church. He would then be "all in" until Wednesday.

He insisted that if I would only examine him carefully enough I could find a local cause for this illness. Because, from the start, I had told him that he was primarily a frail person with an overly sensitive nervous system, when I found a small cancer growing in his rectum, he crowed over me! He said, "You see; I was right."

I told him we would, of course, remove the little tumor, but much as I would love to cure him, I could not hope to do this with the little operation needed to rid him of the growth. It was "silent" — in other words, not producing any of his symptoms. When he left Rochester, he vowed to return some dayand show me how wrong I was. Four years later he came back and said, "It is lucky for you I am a minister of God with a compulsion to tell the truth. I have to admit you were right, and the removal from my body of *even a cancer* left me just as frail, and sickly, and sensitive to emotion as ever I was."

Often when I see a neurotic and fussy woman with her symptoms all pointing to a constitutional frailness — but anxious to have a big operation performed for a silent diaphragmatic hernia, a silent gallstone, or a small silent "fibroid" of the womb — I remind her of what the wise old Chinese say, that, "One should never call in a tiger to chase away a dog!"

I see many an unhappy woman whose main trouble seems to be that she is married to a man who, while he shows signs of being loving, never learned to love a woman in an "acceptable way;" he never learned to do the many kind and thoughtful little acts, or he never learned that little gifts — if they show thoughtfulness and a remembrance of the loved one's liking for certain things — mean much more than a very expensive gift that was not well chosen.

I remember the wife of a banker who was full of aches and pains for which I could find no physical cause. Then, as I so often have to do, I asked, "Why are you so sad?" And she said she thought her husband loved her, but he did it in ways that gave her no pleasure, and sometimes even annoyed her. For instance, after their marriage he left with a florist an order to send her a dozen red roses every Friday. She said, "Perhaps I am wrong to feel as I do, but now, after two years, every time those roses come I feel like screaming and throwing them at him. The trouble is that they bring me no feeling of a thought-taking affection on his part."

To show what I mean by acceptable loving, I remember the great pleasure a patient of mine felt when her husband found a piece of rare Meissen porcelain for which she had long been searching to fill a gap in her collection. He showed real love for her, first, in knowing what she wanted, and then in spending much time searching for it.

After I became well acquainted with the clinical pictures of many syndromes which I came to call "minor equivalents" of psychoses and epilepsy, I found it easy to make many a diagnosis which in my early days would have been an unsolvable puzzle. For instance: one day, in from Paris came a Latin American diplomat who said that on sitting down to a meal, he would go into a "tizzy" in which he would feel as if he were going to die; his pulse would race, he would perspire freely, and he would become nauseated; areas of goose-flesh would appear on his skin; he would tremble all over, and he would hurry to the toilet, fearing that his bowels were about to move.

Because I knew this story, having heard it several times before, I just asked the man who in his family had been mentally odd, and he said he had two close relatives in a mental hospital, two uncles so violent that they were afraid some day they would kill someone, and several "goofy" nieces. When I told him I was satisfied that his nervous storm was his small share of the family curse of jittery nerves, he said he could easily accept this idea because for long he had suspected that he had inherited some of his family's neuroticism. Today, with a much larger experience to draw upon, I would look for an element of epilepsy in this man's type of hot-tempered family; I would get electroencephalograms made, and I would probably find the erratic wave forms of epilepsy.

Early in my medical life I became interested in these odd families in which one member was psychotic or at times insane, and other members had milder nervous or psychic troubles — which looked to me like "equivalents." In 1958 I described 673 of these troubled families in a book called *Practical Leads to Puzzling Diagnoses: Neuroses That Run Through Families.* I wish it could have had some influence on the thinking of American psychiatrists but I fear my thousands of collected *facts* were not interesting enough; sexual theories, like those of the Freudians, are so much more fun.

During the years from 1932 to 1946, I was so swamped with practice that often I could not do much research, and this distressed me. But somehow I managed to keep working on a few problems, near-always working quite alone. My records indicate that in my quarter century at Mayo's, I wrote 739 articles, 329 editorials, a few books and several chapters in systems of medicine, as well as finding time to give many lectures.

In 1929, I was made President of the Gastroenterological Association. Five years later, I began to write editorials for the American Journal of Digestive Diseases. And in 1941, I started editing a new journal called simply, *"Gastroenterology".*

Although it means hard work, I like writing editorials; it gives me the chance to call to the attention of many thousands of physicians those advances in medicine which I think at the time have outstanding value and significance.

For a year or more I was on the Governing Board of the Macy Foundation in New York. I was on it long enough to learn how extremely difficult it is to allocate moneys for the purposes of research, with any probability of getting some return on the investment. After seeing most of our grants wasted on applicants who had not previously done much work of value, I decided that the most logical thing to do would be to help only those men who had already done some excellent research, and who seemed to have opened up a good "lead" into a problem.

But even with them, nearly all of our money went down the drain, and brought no results. Even a man like Sir Frederick Banting, after his great success with insulin, confessed sadly to me that he could not get going again, although for years he tried hard to find "the secretion of the adrenal glands."

Incidentally, I was asked to resign from the Macy Board because I objected to our wasting money on those surveys which are so dear to the hearts of many heads of Foundations, but the reports of which, so far as I can learn, are seldom read or studied or used by legislators.

Friends often ask me how I manage to keep getting so much work done, and I say the secret is to keep using those many scraps of time which most of us waste. Always, and particularly when traveling, I have a briefcase with me, and if I have to wait anywhere — even for a few minutes — out comes my work. Naturally, I get much done evenings, and on Saturday afternoons, Sundays, and holidays. I work seven days a week.

Some may say, "But what a dull and stupid life that must be!" Actually, it is a most interesting and satisfying life, because it is the one I like to live. Every so often I take a few days off for a little vacation, perhaps combined with a lecture somewhere. I imagine I inherited my love of work from a very active father and mother. Like my father, I could never just sit and rest. I have always marvelled at people who thoroughly enjoy loafing. It must be a hereditary gift!

In 1928 I published a much enlarged second edition of the *Mechanics of the Digestive Tract,* and in subsequent years I brought out the third and fourth editions which were big quartos with a new title: *An Inductroduction to Gastroenterology.* In 1947 I finished writing the last edition, and since then I have not done much reading in physiology. My interests changed. In 1930, I published *Nervous Indigestion,* and the edition sold right out. Thirteen years later, in 1943, I much enlarged the book and called it *Nervousness, Indigestion and Pain.* This quickly sold over 35,000 copies, and now, rewritten in simpler English, it is going between paper covers to thousands of lay people.

Much of what I got done through the years was done with dogged persistence. If a committee refused me permission to go on with a certain bit of research, of if they refused permission to publish my work, I immediately went at something else.

Along the way I learned never to be dismayed or diverted from my work by the receipt of a highly critical or perhaps abusive letter. To illustrate: in the beautiful medical museum which I started in Rochester, the Director, Dr. Arthur Bulbulian, put in a fine exhibit showing the progressive development in the womb of the human embryo and fetus. When a sex-hating old maid complained, accusing us of showing obscenities and corrupting the children of the land, Dr.

W. J. Mayo was so upset he called me and told me to take the exhibit right out.

I said, "Of course, Dr. Will, I will do what you wish, but why should we be influenced by this one stupid woman and not by the thousands of fine mothers and schoolteachers who each year bring crowds of children to learn from this exhibit something of the origins of human life? Actually, this exhibit is one of the most popular in the whole museum." "You're right," said Dr. Mayo, "Disregard the letter." The exhibit remained in place, and I never heard of another complaint about it.

I learned another valuable lesson about critical letters when I was helping Dr. Bulbulian to build the Mayo Clinic's exhibit at the World's Fair in Chicago. One day my merry friend, Dr. Carey, the physician in charge of the building all of the medical exhibits, came to me much perturbed by a most unpleasant letter he had just received from an official of his school, scolding him for having permitted the showing of a collection of human fetuses — which actually was the most popular exhibit in the whole scientific division of the Fair. As Dr. Carey said to me, "I cannot understand why Bill wrote me that awful letter, because we are old and good friends."

The next time I saw Dr. Carey, he was happy, and said, "Oh, that was all right; my friend had forgotten to tell me that he wrote that letter only so that he could give a copy to the bishop; and the bishop wanted it only to show devout church members that he had already protested against 'the outrage.' "

Many a time since then, when I have received a letter of bitter criticism from some pious woman objecting to perhaps a few words on sex in one of my newspaper columns, I have just chuckled and said to my secretary, "There's a letter that was written for the bishop!"

In the Mayo Clinic one of the things I used to try to teach my assistants was that on those rare occasions when one of them got embroiled with some testy or "difficult" or somewhat psychotic patient, it was because he had taken a dislike to the man or woman, and had shown it. Usually when I went in to calm down and appease the person, I found a good soul who was frightened, or felt he hadn't been treated nicely. All I had to do was to show that I liked him (her); to apologize, and then to see that the person got the best of care, and kindly treatment. Many of those supposedly "ornery" persons whom I saw a third of a century ago are still writing me a sweet note every Christmas; we have been good friends for all these many years.

I have always felt that to the three little Japanese monkeys who "see no evil, hear no evil and speak no evil" there should be added a fourth — the most important one — who will *"think no evil."* When I think no evil of a patient, and especially when I "take a shine to him" he usually likes me. Many a time I have gotten along beautifully, even with a psychotic patient, because I have talked to him much as I would have talked to a loved brother or an old friend. I have gotten along even with paranoiacs by never questioning the fact that they had noted something that had alarmed them; all I suggested was that I, who am not easily alarmed, would probably not have interpreted what they saw or heard as a threat to my safety.

Very satisfying was my experience with the many patients whose life-stories cheered me and warmed my heart — because they showed me what a strong love can make some people do. For instance: I have always admired the understanding and loving kindness of a certain ranch woman who, on discovering that her husband's "business trips" to the city were really dipsomanic debauches, or "lost week-ends," decided to go with him and take care of him. Because she saw so clearly that what he had was a form of mental disease, instead of blaming him and scolding him, she just went aong and sat in his hotel room for several days, reading and knitting, while he lay on the bed, dead drunk. Later, when he would come out of his spell, they would quietly go back to the ranch and take up their usual way of life again.

During my years of medical practice, I learned a number of very helpful "tricks" of diagnosis, such as looking carefully at the patient and sometimes seeing a number of significant symptoms. For example, signs in the face, speech, behavior, or dress often indicate some minor brain damage, usually due to a "little stroke." In 1930, I found that most of my graduate students were reluctant to accept this idea. I have been shocked when a professor of medicine or neurology failed to note obvious brain injury in a patient. It occurred to me that teachers of medicine ought to have a selection of photographs of people with brain injury, and *to* familiarize students with them.

It is very important to not only get a detailed medical history, but also a thorough *family history.* As an eminent neurologist once wrote, "A family history taken carelessly is often of no value." In many cases in which the patient was ashamed of the cause of his illness, I learned about by having him come for questioning every day for a week or more.

A most valuable "trick" was that of asking the spouse or some other close family member if they know what has been causing the patient's disease or discomfort. It is essential in diagnosing the very common "little strokes" to ascertain if the illness came suddenly or at a particular time of day. For example, once when I saw a certain man who was the leading attorney in the city of his residence, I was instantly attracted by his dull and slovenly appearance. And when I was taken by his son into the family parlor, the patient did not look at me or greet me. I marvelled that the man's family doctor, who had a large practice in that city, did not seem to notice the terrible wrongness of his appearance and behavior. I immediately asked the patient's son when the big change had taken place in his father, and he said, "It came when Dad was running the annual meeting of his university. Suddenly he fainted and fell out of his chair! But he picked himself up and managed to go on with the meeting. The next day, however, he had another brief loss of consciousness." I then said to his family doctor, "Obviously, his brain has been damaged by two strokes." But he replied, "Oh, that is foolishness; he has chronic appendicitis and he should be operated on." Needless to say, I was amazed at this senseless diagnosis.

Another such example occurred when one day I met an old and dear fraternity brother, a professor of medicine in a great university. When we met, he would not look at me or stop to greet me; he simply ignored me and walked away. The minute I saw my old friend, I knew that his dull and expressionless face the fact that his clothes were not clean, and that he limped slightly when he had not done so before, all indicated that he had some brain damage. Shortly after, when I met the medical professor who had recently examined him, I asked him when my friend had had the stroke. He said, "No, there has been no stroke. All his tests were normal." A few days later I learned that he had died after a final stroke.

Also very important in many a case is asking the patient to show with the fingers just where the pain is in his or her stomach. One elderly woman with "silent" gallstones, pointed to her left hip-joint! Her son then told me that while crossing an avenue, his mother had been suddenly almost paralyzed. She too had undergone a "little stroke."

Many times I correctly diagnosed an allergic cause of patient's illness when, while he was a week or more away from home, the symptoms disappear. Then it was up to me and the patient to find out what it was at home that had caused the trouble. Usually the patient helped, or even made the discovery himself with what I called "home detective work."

To illustrate: I learned that a sensitive woman, while at Rochester, did not get one of the frequent asthmatic spells which she had in her own home and in her mother's home. She told me that she did not have these attacks when she was in either her brother's or her sister's home. I then got her husband to study the inner walls of those four houses to see if he could find anything amiss in the two "bad" houses. The next day he reported that the "bad" houses had patches of unpainted and unvarnished beaver board. When these boards were varnished, the woman did not complain further of having asthma attacks.

In many cases I suspected a food allergy when a patient, during his stay at Rochester, did not experience the indigestion or dullness of faculties which was so distressing at home. The most remarkable case was that of a very intelligent college student who, when he was first brought to Mayo's, was apparently stupid. But after a few days of staying in a hotel, he became bright and energetic again. We discovered the cause sometime later when some questioning revealed that this dullness occurred whenever he went to visit his devoted grandmother. It seems that she would give him each morning a breakfast consisting of an omelet of five eggs, and this was the culprit!

An interesting case of home detective work was that done by an intelligent farmer who sometimes got a brief spell of asthma. When he had no trouble while in Rochester, I said, "Go home, and keep a record of any unusual activity or eating just prior to having a spell." He phoned me later and said that he had gotten a spell when he had driven into the city. I asked him to drive to the edge of the city and see if he wheezed, and he reported that he did. Then I had him go the same route in a friend's car and then in a bus. In both instances he had a spell, so we concluded that the cause was not connected with either his home or his farm, and that probably something along the highway itself was the cause. Then I got him to drive very slowly along the highway so he might observe what part of it affected him. He reported to me excitedly that the spells were due to a swamp elder bush! After that, by simply using an alternate route, he was "cured."

CHAPTER X

THE DOCTORS MAYO

I always admired Dr. Will Mayo. I had such respect for him that often when I met him on the street my hat was off before I realized what I was doing. He had a distinguished face with piercing eyes and the glance of a man with an iron will. As I looked at him I always had the feeling that he would have been a great leader in any business. There was goodness and honesty and often kindliness in his face; also great purpose and great dignity. There was so much dignity that not even eminent friends in the field of surgery thought of calling him by his first name or reaching out to touch him.

With one look he would seem to see into a man's soul, and to ascertain all he needed to know about him.

He was of medium height, but strongly built as became a man who in college had been a champion boxer. He always stood straight as a soldier, and until the end of his days he walked rapidly with a firm step. He always spoke well and convincingly.

I never ceased wondering how, when he first met me, he knew instantly that he could tell me anything and I would keep it secret as long as he lived. In fact, some of the things he told me I do not feel I should reveal, even today, after his death. As early as the first week or two after I arrived in Rochester, he told me of his concern over the unwise behavior of three members of the Staff, and he even asked my advice about possibly dismissing one or two of them. Imagine what a storm would have been kicked up in the Clinic if I had ever said a word about this! And I hadn't been around the place more than a few days before Dr. Will asked my advice in regard to a successor to a prominent member of the Staff who was retiring. When I suggested a certain man, Dr. Will said, "Send for him."

I marvelled at the quickness with which Dr. Will could make an important decision. One day, around 1931, I suggested to him that we build a medical museum so as to house the many fine exhibits our artists were constantly fashioning for big medical meetings. Instantly Dr. Will said, "A good idea. Take the old four-story school building across the street. Phone our architect in Minneapolis and arrange to have a man here tomorrow at 9 a.m. Find an excellent artist to help you, and go to work tomorrow morning."

Interestingly, that afternoon and the next morning, Dr. Will kept phoning me at two hour intervals to make sure that I had started the project! Luckily, I had found a splendid artist at the Minnesota University and had hired him. I telephoned the architect and also secured the help of Dr. Henry Plummer. The next morning, the four of us went to work.

Dr. Will behaved in much the same way when in 1931 he called me in and said, "Go to Chicago and decide whether or not we should build an exhibit for the World's Fair. The Board of Governors has refused four times to make the exhibit — with good reason, fearing some doctor's bitter criticism — but some of the most eminent physicians in Chicago want us to make it. So go and investigate the matter, and whatever you advise, that will I do." My report to him advised that we should go ahead and build it. Instantly, he instructed me to find a suitable artist and get started on the project. I found Dr. Bulbulian, a dental student who preferred his avocation as an artist. So he and I proceeded to build the exhibit.

I feel I must say here a few words about Dr. Henry Plummer, who was one of the original partners of the Doctors Mayo, and the most unusual character around the Clinic. He was one of the oddest and most absent-minded of men. Many a time — talking to himself — he passed me on the sidewalk, three feet away, without seeing me. At other times he would grab me like the Ancient Mariner, and start talking to me in a monologue for four hours — or as long as I would stay. The difficult feature of these interviews was that I generally came away from one of them with but a vague idea as to what Henry had been trying to tell me. His mind seemed to run on ahead and leave his lips behind to talk by themselves!

One day Henry opened his heart to me and talked more lucidly than he had ever done. He said that none of the original partners, besides Dr. Will, had ever shown any love of planning ahead, directing, managing and building the Clinic. Each day they did their work with patients, and that was that. He it was who had to build laboratories, an X-ray department and most of the machinery needed for the handling of patients and their histories and X-ray films, etc. Henry said he had always felt that he was largely a "hired man" who kept taking over Dr. Will's plans, quietly implementing them, and working out their details. Often, however, if he saw that something like a new building was much needed, he would keep talking to Dr. Will about it until eventually he wore him down and got his permission to go ahead. As Henry said, he marvelled at Dr. Will's lack of any interest in erecting buildings to house the Clinic. In the early years, Dr. Will seemed content to *rent* space, and to get along with terribly crowded quarters. When I first went to work in the Clinic, it was like a rabbit warren, with burrows leading out into the second floors of the buildings on the block.

One day, I was much surprised when Henry told me that he had always felt, just as I did, the loneliness of a man who "did not belong." As Henry said, we both had had to suffer for much the same reason: neither of us had ever settled down into any well-known "groove in the machine." He had to do much building, while I did research and lecturing and writing. As he said, this sort of non-conformity upsets people, most of whom love a well-ordered, well-known, and unvarying routine.

Obviously, Henry's extremely useful and constructive activities had been very different from those of any other man in the Clinic, and hence he "did not belong to the gang." Also, as often happens with a man who has a touch of genius, he had none of the play-habits or petty vices of the crowd; he had no cronies, and all of this must have made for great loneliness.

I could tell a dozen remarkable and amusing stories about Henry and his extreme absent-mindedness, but instead I will tell a story which will astound his old friends. One day I said to him, "In three weeks Dr. Walter B. Cannon, my dear old professor from Harvard days, will be here, and I am inviting a group of research-minded men to have luncheon with him at my house; will you honor us by coming?" Henry said, "I will be glad to." On the morning of the luncheon I called Henry's secretary to ask her to remind him.

"Oh, no," she said, "he so wants to meet Dr. Cannon, that all by himself, he remembered." And exactly at twelve he walked in!

Once he told me that it can be a great help to a busy man to have a reputation for extreme forgetfulness: it can get him easily out of all sorts of time-consuming commitments!

Dr. Will was the only man I ever stood in awe of, and yet he was easily approachable and very democratic. There were no secretaries sitting outside his office to keep people away. In the early days, when I was on an auto trip with him, and we had luncheon, his chauffeur would sit at the table with Dr. and Mrs. Mayo and their guests. In the Clinic anyone could come up to talk to Dr. Will, and often he would say to the assistant with him, "See that this person gets into the hands of 'so-and-so' " — the specialist that could best take care of the man's problem.

Dr. Will was always very kind to me, sometimes as kind as a father. He was always very appreciative whenever some little honor came to me. He would either send me a kind note, or he would come hurrying up to me in the hall to tell me how pleased he was. Often, to my great surprise, I found that he had read some paper I had written. I never could understand how he found the time to keep in such close touch with what those of us on the staff were doing.

Curiously, Dr. Will was once a bit apologetic to me, apparently fearing that I might think him lazy! When one day, on his big 100-foot Diesel cruiser on the Mississippi River, I came on deck and found him sitting, staring into the water, he said, "I think I am behaving wisely — sitting here, just thinking, because I am figuring how I can strengthen certain weak sections of the Clinic, and wondering how I can improve our public relations with the medical profession. I think I am of more use here, thinking and planning, than I would be at Rochester, operating." And I heartily agreed with him.

I always marvelled at the amount of reading he did. If he liked a book very much he marked it with an *A,* and it remained in his library. If he liked it but did not want to keep it, it was marked *B,* and given to one of his daughters. But if it was marked with a *C,* it went "out."

It was remarkable how closely he kept in touch with what was going on in the Clinic, and throughout the country. He could get by with only four hours of sleep a night. He said that the remainder of the night he just lay quietly and rested and thought. When out to a dinner, he always went home at 9 P.M., if only because next morning at eight he would be operating. He always took a brief nap after luncheon. He would lie back in a chair or on his bed and immediately get 20 minutes of sleep that would keep him going well all afternoon. In spite of all the terrible pressures on him, every day he kept his appointments — right to the minute. I never saw him drink hard liquor, and I never saw him smoke.

Occasionally he gave me a glimpse that showed that the strain of running the Clinic was heavy upon him. He admitted to me that he found it a very lonely job. He explained once how he could not have intimates among the Clinic men without making it seem possible, when a dispute arose, that his decision had been influenced by favoritism. I reminded him of the great Pharaoh Amenemhet, who, when turning over the government of Egypt to his son, Sesostris, warned him that a man in a position of power must live and work in loneliness. As the old King said,

> Fill not thy heart with a brother,
> Know not a friend,
> Nor make for thyself intimates.

This sort of reserve is a good trait for a top executive to have, and it can be beneficial also for relatives that he may wish to place into higher positions.

One day, shortly after arriving at the Clinic, some of my friends saw how kind Dr. Will was to me, and one of them said, "You should be glad that he does not make you the head of a department or something like that, because it would no doubt cause trouble for you."

Dr. Will once put a nephew who was not particularly outstanding into a position of authority. The poor fellow came to me and said that he knew many men in the Clinic were jeering at him, and it was an unhappy situation for him. He asked my advice about whether or not he should get Dr. Will to excuse him from the position. I managed to help him to do it without hurting Dr. Will's feelings. Later, Dr. Will admitted to me that he realized that he had only distressed the man he had wanted to help.

He told me how hard it was on him, on rare occasions when he had to dismiss someone from the Clinic. He confessed that at such times he would leave town for a while until the storm had blown over. One of the oldest members of the staff told me that, in the early days, if a Clinic man was misbehaving, Dr. Will would call him in and give him a stiff talking-to. But in my day he used a special technique for admonishing a man without causing him to lose face or to have to remember a painful interview. Dr. Will would send the man's best friend to him to say something like, "I just saw the Old Man and I judged from what he said that he'd be much happier if you would do thus and so (or would stop doing something or other)." I know that when, in 1927, Dr. Will decided that I must spend my afternoons seeing patients instead of doing research, he did not say anything to me. He sent my best friend Dr. Leonard Rowntree, who said, "Walter, I just saw Dr. Will, and you take my advice — you do right now what Dr. Will wants you to do." And I did it.

Only a few of the oldest members ever called him "Will." The rest of us called him "Dr. Will," much as in Spain a prominent man is called Don Luis or Don Jose. Once he remarked to an intimate that he would like to have more people call him Will, and another time when he saw an old friend put his arm around Dr. Charlie's shoulders, Dr. Will said, "No one ever did that to me." But then, he added, "If anybody did, I don't suppose I'd like it."

Dr. Will must have been one of the country's best executives, because he built the world's greatest Clinic so quickly. When choosing new staff members, he had an uncanny skill.

One of the many things I liked about Dr. Will was his fondness for giving a man a kindly pat on the back when he had done a fine piece of work. He was big enough to give a man credit and to do it generously, and while the man was still living! He would say, "An ounce of taffy is worth a pound of epitaphy."

No one of us is perfect, however, and sometimes I saw Dr. Will do things which seemed to me to be unwise. For instance, he told me he believed in "throwing a new man into a department" without first discussing the matter with the head of that department. I remember a day when he telephoned Dr. Hugh Cabot and invited him to join the kidney and bladder division of the Clinic. How strange it was that Dr. Braasch, who for years had been head of that section, was not consulted in the matter, and was not even told that the new man was coming!

Naturally, such behavior on Dr. Will's part was disturbing to many of the men on the staff, and this made it extra rough on the new man coming in. Sometimes, when his welcome was not warm, the man would wish that Dr. Will would say a few words in his behalf. But Dr. Will told me he would never openly help a newcomer. He would say that if the new man succeeded in holding his own and perhaps fighting his way to the top, all well and good: he would have justified Dr. Will's faith in him. If he went under, that was just too bad, and he could leave.

I have known other top administrators who, like Dr. Will, would not say a word to help a man who was having serious troubles with his associates — men who had never desired his entrance into their department. Such behavior on the part of a top executive has always saddened me, especially when it has led to the expulsion from the group of one of their ablest men. I can see, however, that an administrator does not care to reprove a pack of small men who are tryng to pull down a big man. The Chief knows that he has to keep the peace with the members of his group, and hence, often, he allows his ablest man to be harrassed, blocked, and perhaps driven out of the university, company, or clinic. I have seen it done many times and in many places.

Dr. Will might not come openly to the rescue of a man in trouble, but he might call him to his office for a few words of cheer. Thus, when in 1927 it came to Dr. Will's attention that I had become fed up with some of the opposition that had arisen against me and my work, and I was thinking seriously of leaving, he sent for me and was kindness itself. He said, "Haven't you learned yet that if a man ever does anything unusual, or fine, or worthwhile, or if mentally or spiritually he raises his head up above the level of the crowd, a few men are surely going to take a crack at it? That is human nature. *It has always been that way in the past, and it will always be that way in the future.* Hence it is that, early in life, every hard-driving man like you should learn to take such attacks in his stride. Don't be bothered or upset. Just continue on your way, satisfied that what you are doing is right.

"Actually," he went on, "when I throw a new man into a section, hoping thereby to put a more vigorous life into it, to give it a better national standing, or to get more research out of it, if within a couple of months some of the men in that group do not come running to me to say, 'Stop him, it looks as if he is going to take over my job and add it to his,' I know I have made a mistake, and have put in the wrong man.

"The thing you must do now is to go out and grow a thick skin. God knows I had to do that once. When Charlie and I proposed to give $1,500,000 to the University of Minnesota for a Foundation, a number of the most prominent doctors in the State — men who we had always thought were our friends — went into the Legislature and fought us bitterly, trying to have the gift refused. No, this little ruckus you have run into just proves to me that you are 'stirring the pool,' and that is what I brought you here to do."

Only on a few rare occasions did I ever hear Dr. Will express contempt for any man, and then always it was because he had discovered that the man was not honest.

Some of the men in the Clinic thought that Dr. Will was sometimes too much of a dictator, but I greatly sympathized with him in his dislike of arguing at length about some inconsequential matter, or of waiting for one or two committees to pass upon it. He liked to get from someone the essential facts about a problem, and then to give a quick decision.

Twice Dr. Will remarked to me that as he grew older he had less and less stomach for fighting, and he got to craving peace, which did not always come easily. I marvelled that many of the doctors on the Staff would run to him and demand that someone be stopped from doing something or other. It never would have occurred tome to do such a thing. One day I remarked to one of my associates that I had invited my dear friend Professor Alfred Barclay of Cambridge University, one of the great research men of England, to come over for a visit and to use my X-ray movie machine for some researches he wanted to carry out. The next day my associate confessed to me that he had run to Dr. Will to protest strongly against Barclay's coming. He said he feared Barclay would overshadow him!

One of the things that I greatly admired about the Mayo Clinic was that approximately thirty percent of the patients who came to Mayo's had very small incomes, and most of those people were therefore not bothered with a bill. Dr. Will told me that himself.

In my day, it never occurred to me to charge a doctor, a doctor's relative, a nurse, a minister, a priest, or a nun. Today, they do get charged of course, but I understand that often Medicare pays their bills.

Dr. Will was one of the kindest men I knew. When one of the Clinic men lost his health so completely that he could never work again, Dr. Will saw to it that the mortgage on his house was paid. When another man died in his early fifties, leaving his finances in bad shape, Dr. Will ordered that his widow be cared for and his children's college education be provided for. One day as Dr. Will was going into the bank, he saw a young man coming out of the president's office looking very discouraged and sad. Dr. Will asked the president, "What's the matter with our friend who just went out?" And the banker said, "He wanted me to lend him a lot of money to buy a hotel, but he has no security."

Dr. Will said, "Look, I often go into that man's late uncle's hotel, and there I find him taking the kindest care of his guests. A man who works that hard, and with that kind of friendliness, cannot lose. So, make out out a note for whatever he needs and I'll sign it." Dr. Will was right as usual. The man, Mr. Kahler, built the finest hotel in Rochester and succeeded eminently. Not surprisingly, he also became a close friend of Dr. Will's, and often went on trips with him.

An example of Dr. Will's thinking was revealed to me shortly after I started work at the Clinic. Perhaps three weeks after I had arrived he called me to his office.

"You still must have some strong impressions about this place. What things do you think are very wrong with the Clinic? Where are we weak?"

I said that my first surprise was that, with psychosis one of the commonest diseases in the world, the Clinic had no department of psychiatry.

Dr. Will said, "Yes, that is a grave defect, but I have always been afraid of putting in such a department because it might get so big as to be unwieldy and perhaps too costly. Also, I am afraid that if I employ a number of psychiatrists, you internists may want to send all your 'neuros' to them. Obviously, you cannot do that. Every one of you in every specialty must take care of your own nervous patients." And I agreed that this would always have to be so.

I told Dr. Will that another department we could not much longer do without was one of statistics. All of our millions of data should be put onto punch cards — which could then be run rapidly through an *IBM* machine. Dr. Will agreed that there was a need for this, but he warned me that most of the oldtimers around the place were not research-minded and distrusted statisticians. If we were to employ one, he would have to be only a "hired man" who would never be allowed to do more than get out figures for use by some Staff member who planned to write a paper.

Later, I got Dr. Henry Plummer interested in the project, and eventually he wangled the necessary appropriation for a fine statistical department.

But even Henry Plummer was hostile to the idea of turning a statistician loose in the place. My friends in the Clinic, from Dr. Will down, warned me never to make any statistical studies myself. They assured me that any such work would get me into hot water. I didn't take their advice, so I got into hot water all right! I felt then like reminding Dr. Will that in 1900, the father of statistics, Karl Pearson of the Galton Laboratory of London, was warned by the Council of the Royal Society to keep his mathematical methods of analysis out of the field of Biology

— or else! As a result, he had to found his own journal *Biometrika,* in which to publish the many papers that came out of his busy laboratory.

But I must emphasize the fact that I encountered this distrust of statistics some 50 years ago, when the science was new and when the old-timers around the place (now all gone to their reward) were men who in their college days had had no training in scientific research, and hence had little if any interest in it. Naturally, many of them had that dread of new things which most of us human beings always have. This sort of resistance was not limited to the Mayo Clinic. Almost everywhere I went — into many a great hospital or university Clinic — I found the older surgeons fearful of letting anyone check up to see what had been the actual results of their operations — particularly on the stomach. They seemed to dread what a statistician's "follow-up" studies might show.

I tried to show some of these surgeons — friends of mine working here and there throughout the country — that by holding back all information they were not fooling anyone. We internists knew approximately what their results were, and we did not like them. In those early days, about the only two surgeons who talked frankly with me about the need for getting more useful types of operations for duodenal ulcers were my good friends, Dr. Frank Lahey of the Lahey Clinic in Boston, and Dr. Alfred Ochsner of the Ochsner Clinic in New Orleans.

In 1920, Dr. Will Mayo, having come to see that the original "surgical partnership" had become large and unwieldy, and that it needed all types of specialists, brought in Dr. Leonard Rowntree, a very fine organizer and professor of medicine from the University of Minnesota. By the time I arrived in Rochester in 1926, Dr. Rowntree had already done a splendid job, and had brought into the Clinic many top-flight men. Rowntree built laboratories in a wing of St. Mary's Hospital, where he grouped around him a number of promising young investigators. (After a few years, these men were heading departments of their own in the Clinic-men like George Brown, E. V. Allen and Philip Hench.)

The coming of new men into the place caused tensions to build up, particularly in the "old-timers" who had never done much writing or lecturing. A few felt, and justifiably so, that they had been so swamped with clinical work that they had never had time for research, writing, and lecturing. Some of these staff members resented the fact that a few men — like me — were called upon to lecture every month — all across the States, leaving the clinicians in Rochester "to earn the money."

Naturally, this feeling of resentment of the oldtimers against the newcomers flared up when, with the coming of the financial crash of 1929, the Clinic became a bit short of cash. When Dr. Rowntree's labs were closed, he became so angry that, even though Dr. Will tried to placate him by offering to increase his salary, he left the Clinic and went to Philadelphia.

I felt that Dr. Will could have greatly reduced the nervous tension at Mayo's by simply telling the research men that he could give them back their laboratories as soon as the financial situation eased up enough to do it; but I never heard him say it.

One day he told me that he was tired of all the arguing and fighting. He said, "I am growing old, and now I want peace. You researchers must not expect me to do your fighting for you any longer." That left me with the impression his sympathy was with the "non-researchers" rather than with the "researchers." But with the return of national prosperity, most of those involved in research got back their laboratories. I did not get mine back because in the intervening years I had gotten very interested in certain rare diseases, and I wished to continue my work. I am happy to say however, that the last time I went through the Clinic buildings, I found many splendid laboratories with expert technicians manning them.

During Dr. Will's last years, he asked me several times to spend a good deal of my time trying to teach the Fellows to do research. But much as I would like to have pleased him on this score, I had to tell him that I was convinced that the only person who is likely to do worthwhile research work is one born with the tendency to be curious, and with a strong desire to get answers to the questions that might come to him.

To show what sort of errors can occur when a physician is not curious and careful, one day my assistant asked me to see a woman patient, age thirty, who had a gallstone that he recommended be operated on. On finding that she had no symptoms indicating gallstones, I vetoed the idea of having her operated on. What excited my curiosity in her case was the brief note in the woman's record that at the age of eighteen she had had a nervous breakdown. That statement had evidently not interested my assistant, but it interested me, and called for more information. Upon asking what shock had brought on the breakdown, she said it was the realization that she was a lesbian and that she could never truly love a man, and she would therefore never have a beau, a husband, children or a happy home. Then I learned that what had caused her to feel her present unhappiness was the loneliness that came when her relationship with another lesbian had suddenly broken up. By talking to her for a while with much sympathy, I was able to relieve her of her unnecessary anxieties.

On a few occasions Dr. Will discussed with me the desperate efforts he was having to make in order to keep journalists and science writers from writing up the Clinic. He knew so well that if an article were published, hundreds of doctors would jump to the conclusion that we had paid for the "advertising," and would be angry in consequence.

One day I saw a man taking pictures in the Clinic building, so I asked him what he was doing. He said that he was getting pictures for an article on the Clinic.

He cheerfully went with me to meet Dr. Will, and when Dr. Will found that the article was to be published in one of America's finest lay journals, he rang up the Editor. When the Editor said that he had already paid $2,000.00 for the article, Dr. Will told him that he would send a check for that amount that very afternoon! And so the article was not published. Another editor later refused to let us off and published an article on Mayo's. Oh, how we were cursed as "damned advertisers!" I am happy to report that the world has improved on that score; three years ago, Victor Cohn, a fine writer, wrote a series of articles on the Clinic, and this time the place was not much cursed.

I was surprised and pleased when one day Dr. Will told me how enthusiastic he was about an article I had written on a simple and economical nonsurgical treatment for duodenal ulcer — with the patient up and about and doing his work. For years, every medical man was supposed to do as Dr. Bertram Sippy for so long had taught: to put every ulcer patient in the hospital for a month. So far as I can remember, I was the first man to come out and say frankly that since more than half of the patients so treated would soon have a flare-up of their old ulcer symptoms, why should we put them to such great expense? Why not let them stay on their job, taking the extra food between meals that would keep most of them comfortable?

Dr. Will said to me, "Many men in medicine fail for lack of a social sense. They do not think of trying to save the patient heavy expense. I see from this article of yours that you have plenty of social sense, *and I like that.*"

One highly significant fact that shows how the physicians and surgeons in Rochester really felt about the operations for duodenal ulcer was that in all my 25 years at the Mayo Clinic I can remember only one of the many menbers of the Staff with an ulcer who was operated on, and he was driven to it late in life by a complication.

One of the things which made the Mayo Clinic possible was Dr. Will's good sense in never interfering in the personal lives of his men. He had some few on the Staff who were very "good" and very religious, and he had others who never went to church. He had men who were excellent husbands, and he had a few who were involved in scandals. He had some who were teetotalers, and some who spent every evening drinking. I admired him much because he did not expect all of us, when off duty, to be angels instead of men.

Sometimes, also, when he probably disagreed with what one of us was saying in public, and even when doctors were writing in to demand that the speaker against the partyline be muzzled, or squelched, or fired, Dr. Will would not interfere with the man's freedom of speech. But I strongly suspect he would have been much happier if the man had first asked if he might take a certain stand, or make a certain statement that would cause the Clinic to be attacked by physicians.

We all know the old saw that no man is a hero to his valet. But Dr. Will was so fine that Louie West, his old chauffeur, once told me that in all his years of traveling around the country with his Chief, he never had had from him an impatient word. Also, Dr. Will's secretary of many years, Mrs. Nora Guthrie, once told me that the longer she worked for

Dr. Will the more she admired him. She and Mrs. Mellish, our chief Editor for several years, were two people around the place who had the strength of character sometimes to say to Dr. Will, "You should not do that."

Dr. Will was a great man and I am the better for having known him. Like all great men, he had a few failings and he made a few mistakes. What was very remarkable was that he could confess to some of these.

That Dr. Will was the "Boss" around the place was evident when occasionally he would reverse a decision of the Board of Governors without bothering even to notify them that he had changed his mind. A few times during the years when a man on the Staff kept rocking the boat, Dr. Will would go ahead, apparently on his own, to dismiss the fellow. He would call the man in and say, "I have an idea that you would be happier working by yourself," and that would be that.

These difficult decisions were made apparentlywithout worrying about what the Board of Governors, or the men on the Staff, would think or say. But when it came to certain matters on which the old-timers felt strongly, Dr. Will seemed to spend much time feeling his way. Even an autocrat knows that he had better keep the peace with that faction in his organization that contains the greatest number of politically-minded men who will vote together.

That the Chief realized the limitations of even his great power around the place became evident to me when once I said, "Dr. Will, can anyone today justify the putting of carbolic acid on the stump of the amputated appendix, and then alcohol? Isn't that a sheer waste of time?" "Yes," said Dr. Will, "it is a silly relic of our ignorance of 40 years ago." I asked, "Why, then, don't you tell the surgeons here to stop doing it?" "No," he replied, "I would not even try. I couldn't stop the practice."

Another time I asked Dr. Will, "Why, when we give a hypodermic injection, do we dab the skin with alcohol? We all know that in a moment it cannot kill any germs: all it does is to waste a gauze sponge and some alcohol." "You are perfectly right," said Dr. Will, "But you try to stop the practice;" and I had to admit that it will probably never be stopped.

On another occasion I said to Dr. Will, "Isn't it awful that the nurses wake a terribly tired postoperative patient at five A.M. to wash her face, at six to take her temperature, and at seven to give her her breakfast. How much better if the poor soul were allowed to get some much-needed sleep." "Yes," said Dr. Will, "This early waking of people is a barbarous, heartless, and senseless practice, but, again, you just try to stop it!" Apparently, someone did stop it because when in 1960 I was operated on in the Methodist Hospital, the nurses let me sleep until seven or eight.

I used to wish, as did Dr. Will, that we could hammer into the heads of all our students the fact that there is much more to surgery than a brilliant operative technique. A fine surgeon will know when *not to operate,* and then, if he has great honesty and devotion to the best interests of his patients, he will not operate. He won't operate even when he knows that his "knife-happy" competitor next door will take on the job.

Dr. Will could be a clever internist if he wanted to be. He told me how once when he was on a vacation in Miami, a millionaire there kept insisting that he come and treat him for an attack of painful palpitation that woke him every night at 3 A.M. and scared the life out of him. No one had been able to help the fellow. Dr. Will kept refusing to prescribe, saying he was a surgeon and on vacation. But finally, to get rid of the man's importunities, he gave him a powerful barbiturate and said, "Set your alarm for 2 A.M.; take this medicine, and then go back to sleep." The man did as he was told; by 3 A.M. he was sleeping so soundly he did not wake, and that was the end of his "heart disease!"

Typical of Dr. Will's ability was the way in which he once saved the life of a bullfighter who had been gored in the ring and was rapidly bleeding to death. The bull's horn had entered the front of the man's thigh and had gone up under his skin to the groin, where it had torn a hole in the big artery which supplies the limb. When the doctor on duty in the operating room under the bull ring could not find the artery to clamp it, he begged Dr. Will (who had been taken to the bullfight by friends) to come down and help him. Dr. Will told me that when he came into the room and saw that the doctor was trying to clamp the artery by blindly poking a long "hemostat" up through the tunnel in the thigh, he picked up a scissors, slit open the top of the tunnel, and in a few seconds had clamped shut the hole in the blood vessel!

Dr. Will often urged me never to utter a word of criticism of the medical profession. But much as I respected his wisdom in most matters, on this point I could not agree. I have always been much impressed with the fact that 150 years ago, when a "scrappy" English physician named Thomas Wakley founded one of the world's greatest medical journals — the *London Lancet* — every week he lashed out at the bad, selfish, unfair, and stupid practices in British Medicine of that time. Naturally, the London specialists struck back at him as hard as they could, but the rank and file of the profession gradually came to see the value to them of what he was doing, and in the end he won out.

My personal experience has led me to believe that when able and idealistic doctors hear a fellow physician speaking out against some bad practice in medicine they admire him for his courage. They know he is doing an unpleasant job that has to be done sooner or later by someone, and they are glad he is doing it.

I have always said to my friends, "We all know there are some bad practices in medicine, and there are a few 'bad actors' with an M.D. degree. Wouldn't it be better, then, for us to try to clean up the mess in medicine ourselves — rather than to wait for a senatorial committee to do the work?"

One of the kindest and most reassuring letters I ever received came from Dr. John C. Brougher, who wrote that to him constructive criticism of doctors is an indication of the critic's high respect for medicine as a profession. He realized that when a doctor criticizes a bad medical practice it is only because he so loves medicine that he wants to see the practice of it grow better.

Dr. Osler, who was one of the kindest and most generous of physicians, could not close his eyes to "the lapses and mistakes wich are inevitable in our work." He sometimes spoke unhappily of the physicians who labor only for money, or who, throughout a lifetime, fail to keep up-to-date. He used to speak sadly of those many young doctors who, after graduation, "die a mental death, and come away, stillborn from college."

In spite of all my criticism of certain practices in medicine, I still feel much as did the great Dr. Langdon-Browne, when he wrote, "Despite some disagreeable eddies and unsavory backwaters, medicine's main stream runs clear, and sweeps onward with a gathering impetus."

In 1939, cells from a malignant ulcer in Dr. Will's stomach had grown up into the glands of his neck. He got his old associate and friend Dr. George Eusterman to examine them and asked, "What do you think?"

George's eyes filled with tears, and he said, "I guess they must be metastases (daughter growths)." Dr. Will said, "Don't take it so hard, George. I've lived long enough, and I am perfectly ready to go."

Dr. Will used to say that he wanted very much to go before he became a forgotten "has-been." That he could not face.

When he saw that death was approaching he sent for the few persons with whom he had had conflicts of opinion and perhaps harsh words, and asked for their forgiveness and the return of their old friendship. I chatted with Dr. Will the day before he died. He was badly jaundiced, but his mind was as clear as ever it was. I guess he felt the need to talk to many people because, in those last days, he sat under a tree in his front yard, where many passers-by stopped to visit with him.

He went suddenly, with his mind clear, still making wise plans for the future of the Clinic.

As many people know, Dr. Charles H. Mayo was very different from his brother. They were different in appearance, in temperament and in interests. Dr. Charlie was less awe-inspiring than Dr. Will, but this had its advantages; one could come closer — mentally and spiritually — to Dr. Charlie, and one could feel an affection such as one could not easily feel for Dr. Will.

I had much affection for Dr. Charlie, and I think he sensed it. He knew also that I always loved it when he came up to me to tell me one of his funny stories. Dr. Charlie always seemed to me to be much like Will Rogers, with much of Rogers' combination of wisdom and humor.

So far as I know, Dr. Will had no hobby besides the Clinic and his cruiser on the Mississippi River; but Dr. Charlie loved farms, of which he had several — all stocked with good cattle and horses.

Although Dr. Charlie was shrewd, with much good "horse sense," so far as I could learn he never had any desire to carry the heavy administrative burdens of the Clinic, and I much doubt if his talents ran in that direction. Many people, because of their affection for Dr. Charlie, tried to foster the idea that he was just as much a builder of the Clinic as was Dr. Will. I imagine that in the early years he worked as hard as Dr. Will did — seeing patients, operating on them, and building up the practice. But in the later years, or certainly after I joined the Staff, it was obvious that Dr. Will was carrying most of the burden of administration.

Friends of Dr. Charlie told me that he liked to live for the day — enjoying life with his loved ones about him. It was Dr. Will who spent most of his time planning far ahead for the Clinic. I never thought of blaming Dr. Charlie for not caring to do this sort of thing, if only because I could not have done it myself. With all my strong affection for Dr. Charlie, his son Dr. "Chuck," and his daughter Louise, I never could see any sense in stirring up an argument as to who had had most to do with building and running the Clinic.

Fortunately, in many a situation like this, two very different partners can get along comfortably, as Dr. Will and Dr. Charlie did — accepting the fact that their interests and their abilities are different. What is sad sometimes is that their women-folk and close friends will get into an argument as to who is the better man. I greatly honored Dr. Charlie for cheerfully having lived a life which was not the one he would have chosen if he had been left to himself. Actually, one day Dr. Will, in one of his moments of great frankness, said to me that he knew that with all the many demands that he had made on his younger brother, he had caused him often to live a life that was not quite congenial to him; and for this he was sorry.

Dr. Will was probably enough of a psychiatrist to realize that it is not easy for a home-loving and farm-loving man to live and work alongside a dynamic, hard-driving, very successful, and very famous older brother. Fortunately, Dr. Charlie seemed never to feel any jealousy. He always seemed full of good nature, good sense, and good humor. I never saw in his behavior or heard in his speech any sign of resentment against his brother, even when Dr. Will made an important decision without consulting him. Two of the oldest secretaries in the Clinic and one of Dr. Charlie's oldest and closest friends all told me that if there was any big difference of opinion between the brothers, Dr. Charlie was always willing to let Dr. Will have his way.

On one occasion I personally discovered how unwilling Dr. Charlie was to get into a fight for what he wanted to do. He had become so keen to have me go on a good-will speaking tour to the medical centers of South America that, when I got back from a trip, I found he had my tickets all bought and ready for me. Then, one of my friends who thought *he* should be the one to go — although he could not lecture in Spanish as I could — raised such a fuss that, although it must have been embarrassing to Dr. Charlie to let me down, he gave in. He said not a word to me; I said nothing, and the matter was just dropped. No one went.

Fortunately, Dr. Charlie always stood resolutely by his brother, even when one day Dr. Will had to dismiss one of Dr. Charlie's sons-in-law. One of the finest things that Dr. Charlie ever did was to tell the Staff right then that whatever happened, he would always stand with his brother. When Dr. Will came home from a trip and heard this, the tears came to his eyes, and he turned and walked away.

Right after these events, Dr. Will got Dr. Charlie to go with him to the annual meeting of the American Medical Association, supposedly so that everyone would see how close they were.

Dr. Will must often have consulted his brother about problems that came up in the Clinic. Many a time, as I passed by the two men, I heard them talking earnestly together. But also, as I stated elsewhere, occasionally I saw Dr. Will make a decision without discussing the matter with anyone — not even Dr. Charlie or the Board of Governors. On several occasions, even after the Board had repeatedly taken a stand against some action, Dr. Will — on his own — would reverse the Board's action.

In Dr. Will's later years, in order to be as fair as he could be to his brother, he never got up to speak before an audience without beginning with the statement that Dr. Charlie was equally responsible for everything that had ever been done and that then was being done in the Clinic.

I loved Dr. Charlie's kindliness and humanness, and his delightful sense of humor. It was much like the droll and very wise humor that his son "Chuck" has. Dr. Charlie never impressed me as being as much of a reader as his brother was, but I suspect he knew better how to live a happy life, surrounded by his devoted wife and his children and good friends. I have often heard that he was a wonderful father to his children, and that at 10 P.M. each evening his sons would walk over to the big home and bid their parents good night.

On the lecture platform Dr. Charlie generally put aside his manuscript, and started telling delightful stories. One that I loved was about the voluntary fire company which, in the old days, used to run to fires pulling a hose cart. When the captain became old and rheumatic, the company elected a new Chief, and decided to have a big celebration in the Armory, at which time they would present the retiring Chief with a gold-headed cane. For six weeks the old captain and the new one met every night to practice their "extemporaneous" speeches of delivery and acceptance. Finally the great night came and the Armory was full of people. The young captain got up and started on his speech, but at the end of two sentences he got stuck. After an agonizing period of looking at the floor and the ceiling, he began again at the beginning. Again he got stuck, so again he started. This time, when he got stuck, he just said, "Here, take your goddamned old cane!"

I remember a time at a huge medical meeting when there had been much acrimonious debate about something or other. Then Dr. Charlie got up, and with a short funny story he showed the doctors what they should agree on. They roared with laughter, and that was the end of the argument.

Dr. Charlie once told me about a farm boy who had brought up a calf. Eventually the animal got so big it dragged the boy around, and he was glad when he could steer it a bit. Dr. Charlie said that that was the way he and Dr. Will felt about the Clinic. He and Dr. Will once told me that in the early days they thought of the organization as just a partnership, but soon everyone began to call it a clinic.

I often saw Dr. Charlie show much wisdom with patients. One day when a half-crazy man became insulting, Dr. Charlie just walked out of the room. When the colleague with him said, "Why didn't you give that fellow the dressing-down he deserved?" Dr. Charlie said, "One damn fool in a room is enough."

Typical of Dr. Charlie was the story he told me once of a decidedly hypochondriac, but otherwise normal, man who insisted that his perfectly good kidneys weren't working well. Dr. Charlie told him to go and eat a watermelon and that would cure him. Later, when the fellow returned to say he was no better, Dr. Charlie asked, "Where did you buy the melon?" "From Jones' grocery." "Oh," said Dr. Charlie, "there's where you went wrong. You should have gotten it from Smith's, across the street." Dr. Charlie loves fun like that, and often his patients joined in the laugh and felt much better for it.

One day when another hypochondriac patient asked if he should sell the business and move to the Southwest, Dr. Charlie said, "That might be a good thing to do. I'm trying to remember its name . . . there is a town down there so salubrious that they had to shoot two men in order to start the cemetery! You ought to go there."

Dr. Charlie taught me a very helpful trick in diagnosis which, many a time since, has gotten me out of a tight spot. He said, "Whenever you cannot guess what is wrong with a man, just ask his wife and she'll tell you what it is." It is remarkable how often I have found this to be true. When a stout jolly farmer came complaining of spells of violent nausea and I couldn't find anything wrong with him and was stumped, I remembered what Dr. Charlie had said. Turning to the wife, I asked her what was bothering the man. She said angrily, "I don't know why he comes here to waste our money. He knows darn well what's wrong with him. He gets nauseated when he goes on a binge of chewing tobacco and swallowing the juice!" When I asked the man if his wife was right, he grinned sheepishly and said, "Yes, but I hoped you'd find something else, so I could go on chewing!"

Another time, Dr. Charlie used this technique to make a most remarkable diagnosis. For 10 days I had studied the illness of a farmer's wife who was suffering from a severe and constant diarrhea. When I had to admit that I had no idea what the disease was, the farmer said, "I'd like to see Dr. Charlie." So I went to Dr. Charlie's office with the couple, and quickly told him that all of the tests had failed to give any hint as to the diagnosis. He simply turned to the farmer and asked, "What do you think has caused the diarrhea?" And the man said, "It's them chickens. They got the diarrhie. She nursed them, and then she got it." Dr. Charlie said, "Bring in a few of the sick chickens and we will examine them." They were found to be full of tuberculosis, and when the woman's discharges were examined for tubercle bacilli, there they were — by the million!

One day Dr. Charlie advised a neurotic woman with a lot of hysterical complaints to go to a faith healer. The woman said angrily, "That's a foolish bit of advice." "True," said Dr. Charlie, "but you have a foolish disease!"

CHAPTER XI

1950-1975

In late 1950, I reached the official age limit of 65, and so was retired from the Mayo Clinic. As I was cleaning out my office desk, I received a telegram from the Society of General Practitioners, saying that the editor of their fledgling journal, *G.P.*, had been badly hurt in an automobile accident, and did I know of any way in which they could continue publication. I immediately telephoned that I would be glad to get it out for them, which I did. Shortly thereafter, I became their Editor.

Their business manager, Mr. Cahill, wanted me to be in Chicago, and so I moved there. I located an office and we moved into a nice hotel apartment nearby. On hearing that I had arrived in Chicago, Dr. Bundesen, head of the Chicago Board of Health, requested that I help him to build up a medical clinic. I helped him in this, and I worked there on my mornings for one year. More patients than I could handle came to consult me in my office, so I referred nearly all of them to my friend, Dr. Hyman.

In June, 1951, I resigned from the Editorship of *G.P.*, and as I left my final meeting there I ran into my old and good friend, Jack Cohen of Minneapolis. He said then — as he had said several times before — that he wished I could help him publish his very valuable abstract journal, *Modern Medicine.* Jack's Editor had a stroke the very next morning, and the day after that I was appointed to that position. In addition to this, I was made the Editor of the journal *Geriatrics.* I worked with those two journals until I retired once again in 1975.

In 1951, my old patient and dear friend, C. W. Follett, helped me to

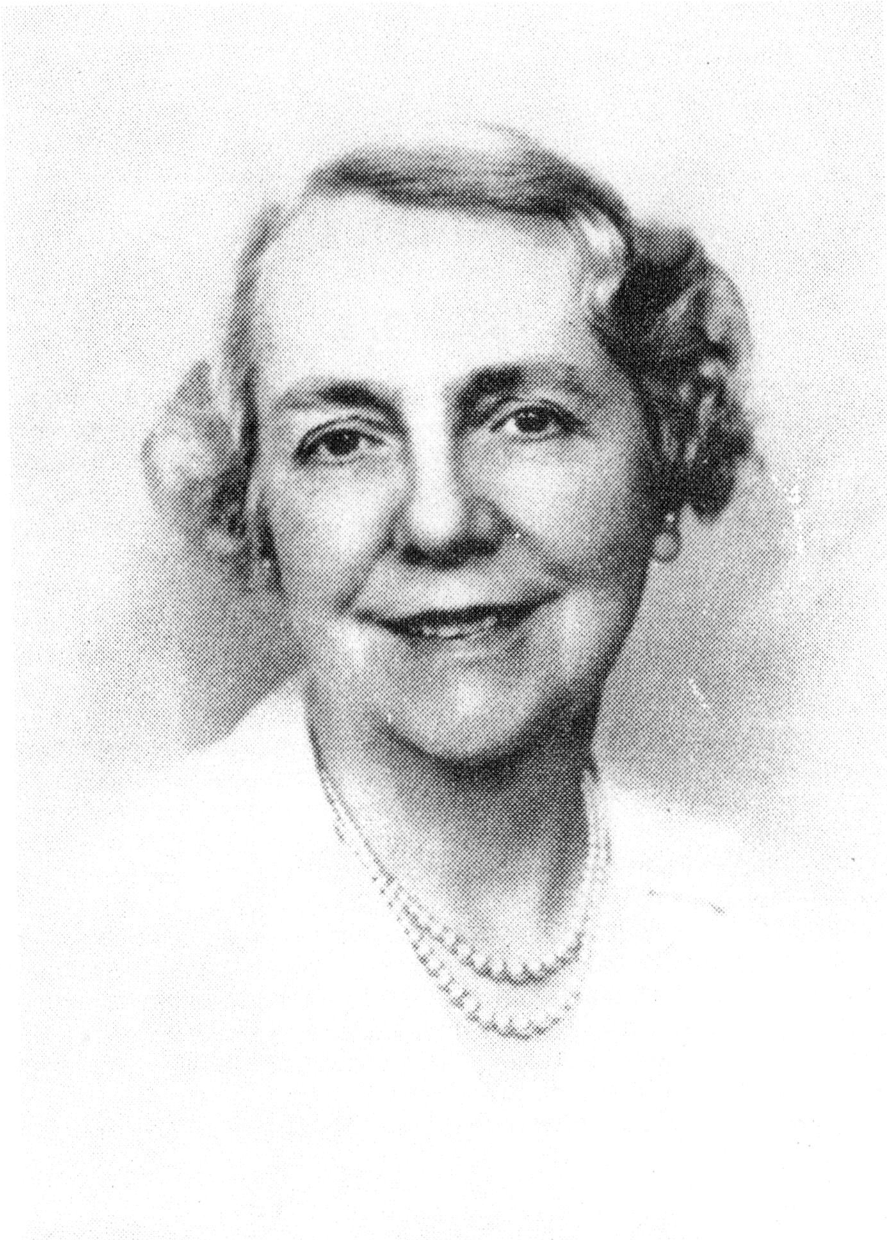

My own dear wife, Harriet

publish some 30 booklets, designed to help laymen understand their diseases; I was to syndicate these booklets in many newspapers.

During the next year and a half, until he died, my friend sold as many articles as I had time to write for him. They were all written in simple English and designed to help laymen to understand their particular problems of disease. Before long, the Register Tribune Syndicate of Des Moines, Iowa, signed me to write four columns a week which were syndicated in some 90 papers in the United States, and 14 more in Canada, Mexico, Brazil, the Phillipines, and Burma.

Naturally, many people wrote to ask me what to do for a stomach-ache, or what type of doctor to get for a bad headache, and all that sort of thing During the first year I received 100,000 such letters. I answered as many as I had time for, and soon had written 30 booklets which the Register Tribune people printed and sold for 25¢ each. They answered many of the more common questions I had received.

I was glad when many of the letters I received expressed great thankfulness for, and appreciation of, my column. Once I heard that a column of mine on eye troubles, in one city, had caused a hundred people to go to an eye specialist; in some cases they went just in time to have their sight saved. Also my column caused a number of mothers to take their diabetic child to a doctor, barely in time to save his/her life.

At first some physicians called me up before the local medical ethics committee to be scolded for suposedly using my columns and booklets to advertise and get patients. But when I showed them that I had so little time left for the practice of medicine that I was sending nearly all of my patients to an able young doctor who was very glad to get them, the committee apologized very kindly, and never bothered me again.

I am happy to say that the relations between doctors and reporters has improved immensely since 1912, when I first started speaking to audiences. Then I was warned by leading doctors never to talk to newspaper reporters; but now, at any big medical meeting, there is a room in which speakers can answer the questions of reporters.

Even before I had gone to Mayo's, I was distressed because I did not know enough to help the many people who came to me worrying themselves sick over sexual problems. Dozens of women came to ask if they should divorce their husbands because they kept asking for some variant of the sexual act. Other women came asking what to do with a son who was sexually attracted more to boys than to girls. In college I had never heard a single lecture on such subjects and, later, much of what reading I had done had left me dissatisfied because so much of the writing was evidently based not on research, but on armchair theories.

Unable to learn of any university where sex was being studied, I went to my good friend Dr. Raymond Pearl, and told him he ought to tackle the job. He agreed that it was a disgrace that so few scientists in America were studying the sexual behavior of men, women, and children, but he said he had so many irons in the fire he could not put in another.

When I heard that Dr. Kinsey had gone to work on the problem, I went to Bloomington, Indiana, and found a fine, dedicated scientist — a man for whom I soon felt a warm friendship. He had seen the need for studies of sex when in his seminars his students kept asking questions which he could not answer.

Dr. Alan Gregg of the Rockefeller Foundation told me that because for so long he had felt the great need for someone to study sexual behavior in man, it had seemed like an answer to prayer when Dr. Kinsey had come in to ask for a grant for the founding of an Institute for sexual studies.

But the results of publishing his studies on human sexual behavior was not so simple. Dr. Kinsey told me of his mental suffering and extreme fatigue caused by his sudden fame. Wherever he went, news writers wanted to interview him. Once, while he was in California, he was able to get a bit of desperately needed rest, not by staying in a hotel, but by arranging to stay in San Quentin Prison, where he was free at last of reporters!

What distressed me when Dr. Kinsey's books appeared was that so many people, even eminent people, attacked him either for not having written in a sweet kindly vein, or for not having been outraged at what he had learned from the thousands of men and women he had questioned. Few people seemed to be able to see that Dr. Kinsey had not written a book to shock, titillate, amuse, or elevate. He was a scientist who had done little more than publish the figures that had come out of his *IBM* machines. He had just reported *what people had said they had done.* He had not felt any need for going on to express strong disapproval of their confessions. It was saddening to me when even some scientific men, who should have known better, could not see that Kinsey had written a book on statistics and not a diatribe on supposed immorality. His book was about what most people do, not what is supposedly *wrong* with what they do.

I often wondered what it was about Kinsey that enable thousands of people to tell him about the most intimate details of their lives. I think they must have sensed what a fine, dedicated man he was — a man who would not "turn a hair" no matter what they told him. Also, he noted down what they told him in a code that was memorized and never put on paper. Hence, if in the future his records should ever get into the wrong hands, no one will ever be able to understand a word of them.

When Dr. Kinsey died in 1958, I lost a good and dear friend.

So often we doctors are expected to be marriage counselors. An unforgettable couple once came to me — he, a tall, austere young New England minister and she, a sweet and loving young thing. When I sensed a tension between them, and saw that this could be the cause of the wife's insomnia, indigestion, and headache, I asked them to tell me what had gone wrong. She said that her husband had the idea that sex was so sinful that it should be tolerated only rarely, and then only for purposes of procreation. She was too affectionate for an unloving marriage of that type. I gave the man a talking-to, and got him to admit that if the good Lord had given us — His children — this strong impulse to be loving, He probably wanted us to use it. The next day I was much pleased to note that when the couple came into my office, they were happy and were holding hands like newlyweds.

Another patient who taught me much about the vagaries of sex was a sweet-faced, lovely, and decidedly feminine Cuban woman of 32, who had never menstruated and had no breasts. For years she had been the well-loved mistress of the man for whom she worked. A careful study, including a surgical exploration of her abdominal cavity, showed that she was as much a male as a female, with tiny glands of both sexes. Because she wanted to go on living as a woman, her very small male organs were removed.

What her case showed me so clearly was that feminine charm and the ability to show warm affection can depend more on something in the brain than on something in the sex glands. I cannot remember ever having learned in books the lesson this woman taught me, and taught me so well I will never forget it. Along the way, I gave her great pleasure by sending my secretary out with her to buy a pair of falsies to put in her bra. With these, she was as pleased as punch.

All my days I have been impressed with what Plato once said, to the effect that in order to be understanding and efficient, a physician should have had the disease he is attempting to treat. I thought of this several times in April, 1960, when X-rays taken at the Mayo Clinic showed a good-sized cancer in my large intestine, and I had to be operated on. The thought then came to me that all my life I had been "dishing out" the diagnosis of cancer,and then I found myself on the receiving end. I was relieved when I experienced it without any undue sense of fear. Fortunately, the operation, which was expertly performed in only forty-five minutes, was very easy on me. My dear friend, Dr. Chuck Mayo and his first assistant, Dr. Kent Cullen, could not have been kinder or more skillful. In three days I was up and walking around. Three weeks later I was back in my office and comfortably at work. Today, seventeen years later, I need not fear that the cancer will return. As I write this, I am hoping that I can keep working hard every day for many more years.

My wonderful and loving wife Harriet died in 1973. I returned to San Francisco to be near my children and other relatives. I am happy to report that even in my nineties, I am still full of enthusiasms. I would hate to be without them — they make life so much more worth living. I love the Greek meaning of the word "enthusiasm". It comes from *en theos* — "a god within." How unfortunate the man or woman who has no god within!

In recent years I have been fascinated by the rapid progress that has been made of late in the field of human genetics.

The following story has always amused me, and it has supported my strong belief in the importance of heredity. Once, when, in a certain city, I spoke about families in which there is much degeneracy, a nice old doctor came up and said, "I know of a queer family down on the mud-flats by the river. One day a patient of mine, a census-taker, told me of a day when he came to a shack there and knocked on the door. When a slattern, stupid-looking girl appeared, my friend asked if her father was home. 'Naw, he's in the penitentiary.' 'Well, is your mother home?' 'Naw, she's at the State Hospital.' 'Have you an older brother?" "Yes, he is in the Reform School.' 'Have you perhaps an older sister?' 'Yes, she works in the red-light district.' 'Well, have you a younger brother?" 'Yes, he's in the medical school at Harvard!' 'Goodness gracious,' said the census man, 'You don't mean to tell me you have a brother who is professor at Harvard?' 'Naw, he's no professor; he has two heads; he's in a bottle of alcohol!' "

Some people who know something of my very busy life, even in my nineties, have asked me if I haven't some hobbies and if there are times when I just rest and relax. So, if I may, I will elucidate a few of my pleasures.

Ever since I was twelve years old I have read a great deal, especially on week-ends, and to me, reading is a restful activity. These days I often have meals with interesting friends, and that too is restful.

On many a week-end I used to take my wife and children on an automobile ride into a suburb or into the hills. During my three years with Dr. Schmoll and my 25 years with the Mayo Clinic, I had month-long vacations during which I often travelled to far places. On twelve occasions, I went for 28-day "High Trips" into the Californian and Canadian mountains with the famed Sierra Club. Travel has always been a pleasure for me. During the 65 years between 1912 and 1977, I have travelled a great deal and over long distances to give lectures or to attend meetings of one or the other society to which I belong.

I also enjoy movies and the theatre. During my forty years in San Francisco and Rochester, Minnesota, Harriet and I saw many movies, and some operas. Of course, we were often entertained by friends, and we entertained in turn.

In the last three years of "retirement" in San Francisco, I have had the joy of visiting my children and their spouses and their splendid children. Some very kindly people in San Francisco and its environs have done much to make life pleasant and interesting for me.

I left Chicago in January of 1975, and retired from the practice of medicine, but I did not retire from the *study* of medicine. I still read several medical journals every month, and continue my reading of books on science. And of course, I have worked very hard over the last year to prepare the manuscript for the "up-date" of my autobiography.

CHAPTER XII

THE FAITH OF A PHYSICIAN

I am reluctant to write here about the puzzlements I have had about matters of religion. The last thing I want to do is to distress my many dear friends who are devout, but still I feel I ought to tell about my efforts to help patients who came to me suffering greatly because they felt that their illness was due to their having inadvertantly offended God.

I should say first that in my youth I tried to be a good church-goer. Later, when I went to college, I often did not go to church because my studies seemed to me more important. When I married Harriet, the very religious daughter of an eminent minister, I not only went to church regularly, but was made a Deacon of the church and found myself "passing the plate." I gave that up when the conservative group in the church dismissed the minister, who was the finest minister I had ever known. I then went to another church because the minister there was so kind and capable. But before long he too was fired. Why? Because when he found that many fine young people would not join the church because they did not want baptism by total immersion, he suggested that they just be "sprinkled" with the baptismal water. This so angered two old retired ministers in the church that they not only threw the minister out of that church, they actually barred him from serving in any California church! After many years of this kind of thing, my devout wife became so annoyed and bored with these conflicts in her church that she quit going. For many years after that she helped the other fine women who entertained lonely soldiers who were passing through Chicago, and in this way expressed her religious feeling.

I too ceased going regularly to church. But I read the Bible from cover to cover and read a number of splendid books about the Bible. Along the way, my religion became devotion to helping my patients with kindness and honesty. In order to help some of my puzzled patients who were worried and ill because they felt that their God must have been angered by something they did, I had to have some form of religion.

For example, one of the finest and most devotedly religious women I ever knew was the daughter of a minister. She herself was a college graduate and the wife of a man who was both a wonderful minister and president of a religious college. All her days she had worked hard to help her church and the church members. I saw her when she was 58, and had just had a bad stroke. She was fortunate in that she soon regained her ability to talk and to walk, but she was left with a peculiar distress in her head. She would ask me, "What could I possibly have done to make God so angry that He struck me down in this way? What mistake did I make?" And I would tell her, 'I am sure that you have not done anything to deserve this, and I am sure that God didn't cause your stroke. All that happened was that a little blood vessel broke in or on the surface of your brain." But she replied, "Look in the Bible, Samuel II, chapter 25, verses 36 through 38, and you will see there a story about a wealthy old grouch named Nabal. One evening, after drinking toomuch alcohol, Nabal said some unpleasant things about Yahweh. His words so angered the Lord that a few days later He 'smoke Nabal' and killed him."

When I studied this and other unpleasant like stories in the Old Testament, I talked about the problems I encountered with a good friend who was a professor of religion. His explanation was that the people of Israel thousands of years ago were not as moral as they are today, and of course their culture was vastly different from ours. In those days, a King could kill prettymuch as he liked without being brought to account for it. The story of King David and Bathsheba comes to mind. David had relations with this beautiful married woman and then arranged to have her husband killed so that he could have her as his wife. The writers of the Bible apparently did not think the story disgusting enough to be left out of a religious text!

Other patients whom I tried to help were some men and women who were very unhappy because their religious spouse refused to engage in much sexual intercourse because he or she believed that God (or St. Paul) was disgusted with it. I managed to talk some of these people out of this ridiculous notion by telling them that if the Creator made sexual intercourse both pleasurable and necessary to the propagation of our race, He cannot regard it in that way. I was glad when, by this argument, I was able to restore to happiness several couples.

A few kindly and concerned priests came to me in a very unhappy state because they feared that once, being weary, they had failed to use all of the necessary words when baptizing a child. They feared that the child would never be saved or accepted in Heaven. I think I helped them by getting them to agree that a compassionate God would never consider punishing everlastingly a perfectly innocent child.

A thing that bothers me about the Bible is that it says some very unpleasant things about homosexual men (but oddly does not mention lesbians). I wish that all of those people who bear hostility against homosexuals would read my little paperback on the subject. They could then see the mass of scientific evidence showing that a homosexual is born with those tendencies, not made into them.

When a devout friend wants me to agree with him that every word in the Bible is God's Word, and therefore always correct, I am tempted to ask him if he agrees with that well-known statement in the Old Testament which says, "Thou shalt not suffer a witch to live." I doubt that there is any psychiatrist practicing today who believes that there is such a thing as a person "possessed by the Devil." Andrew White, the former great president of Cornell University, said in his two volume work, *A History of the Warfare of Science with Theology in Christendom,* that that one sentence about killing witches led to the cruel torture and death by fire for thousands of harmless, if eccentric, elderly women, and even some girls, whose only "sin" was a bit of nervousness, hysteria, or mild psychosis. Fortunately, in the 18th Century laws were passed in England and France prohibiting this barbaric practice.

I have often wondered how people can say that every word in the

Bible is God-given and therefore correct, when in some editions of the Bible, there is a complex list of varients on almost every page. Some words may be more correct than others. I wish all persons who puzzle and argue over many statements in the Bible would read, as I have read, two splendid books by that great student of Biblical texts, Professor Guignebert. After a lifetime of studying the Biblical texts in their original ancient languages, he stated at the close of several chapters that so many errors were made by copyists over the centuries, that we will probably never be able to determine what the original text was.

Some readers may be wondering why I care to live if I am not sure about the rewards that may come with religious faith. My answer is that my happiness has been in helping thousands of the sick and troubled, and trying to make the art and science of medicine a bit better than I found it. Years ago I was helped by reading two autobiographies — one by that eminent physicist, Professor Millikan, and the other by a former high prelate of the Catholic Church, Father Ildefonso, who later called himself John Tettemer.

Strange to say, these two men with such divergent training and background eventually reached the same conclusions: that there are two very different facets to the Christian religion. One is a faith in the simple and compassionate teaching of Jesus, and the other a dependence upon the many fundamentally unprovable theories about the exact nature of God, and theories of the nature of the Holy Family. Theories which for ages have been argued about and fought over bitterly with no profit to anyone.

Professor Millikan said that there are two basic groups of people who profess belief in God but cannot exactly define Him. They are like Zophar or Job in the Book of Job. Zophar asked Job, "Can'st thou by searching, find out God?" And Job replied, "What I did not understand, I uttered: things far beyond me of which I had no knowledge." (Job 42:3)

Father Ildefonso, once a professional theologian and advisor on Church Law to the Vatican, wrote a book entitled *I Was a Monk*. This wonderful man, after a great mental travail, wound up with practically the same religious ideas that Professor Millikan and I have come to. During a long stay in a tuberculosis sanitorium, where he had the time in which to do a great deal of thinking, he, like Job, lost his faith in the power of the human mind to know the Truth and the Ultimate; but he retained his faith in the simple teachings of Jesus of Nazareth. With this change, he felt a release and an uplifting joy. He felt that he had gained a new life and come closer to God.

CHAPTER XIII

THOUGHTS ON THE THEORY OF EVOLUTION

Some readers of this book may wonder why I am putting in a chapter on evolution. The principal reason is that I have been an ardent student of that subject ever since I was in high school. I once had 30 books on Charles Darwin, his family and his work.

Darwin once wrote that as he got older, he lost more and more of his faith in religion. Early in his life, as a student of geology, he learned that the writer (or writers) of the book of Genesis were mistaken when they listed Man as one of the first beings to be put on Earth. I cannot imagine their so listing Man if they had known that the world of plants and animals existed for millions of years prior to the advent of Man, the last and finest of all the living things. But of course the author of Genesis did not know much, if anything, of geology. I recently saw photographs of some tiny fossilized organisms that were found in rock that had been brought up from the bottom of very deeply drilled wells. There the rock strata are very old indeed. (The skeleton of a whale was found recently in the rock of a hill 160 feet above the nearby ocean!) With accurate chemical methods the age of rocks can be measured, and therefore, the age of a fossil or other remnant within that rock can be determined. Geologists know now that certain small skeletons, like those of small fishes, can be very ancient, while those of large animals are found to be of more recent origin.

And then, a few hundred million years ago, some form of human beings appeared. I remember well the day when, in my boyhood, I was impressed by the fact that the lizard I had caught had "hands" with five fingers that looked much like my own. I was impressed too, when I caught a centipede and saw that it had a spine with many segments much like those in my own spine. Such observations taught me a great deal about evolution. I recall vividly seeing in the great biological exhibit in the New York City museum, a series of skeletons, showing clearly that horses had developed from small animals called the Eohippus. I found photographs in a medical journal a few years ago of boys with tails — and I read that in the first year or so of life a human embryo, in its mother's womb, has a tail, which later disappears. There are indications that a type of ulcerated area on a person's neck is the remnants of gills! It is interesting to note also that I once had as a patient a man with five breasts!

After a lifetime of study of animal and human physiology, I still marvel at the complexity of the chemistry that has gone into the making of our bodies, our brains, and the innumerable chemicals which control the workings of our bodies. I marvel also that the chemicals that arrive in the tiny ovum in a woman's womb can make another person who will probably resemble the parents, and may even have the same touch of genius that one of his ancestors had. What sort of chemical combination could have given Mozart, at the age of six, his ability to compose magnificent music?

The fact that the Evolutionary Designer often behaved much like a brilliant engineer is shown by the design of the human eye. The transparent cornea is in front of the globe. Next is a transparent lens with a little iris to regulate the amount of light that passes through it; attached to this is a muscle that will strengthen or weaken the lens so that the person can see near or far. In the back of this mechanism is the retina which is connected to the wonderful brain by a set of nerves. Near the front of the eye is a gland that makes tears that keep the cornea moist and clean. If too many tears are formed, there is an opening that can take them down into the nose. Then there are the muscles that enable a person to look up and down and from side to side, and there are the eyelids that can close and protect the eye from excessive light, and enable us to sleep. What a marvelous and subtle organ!

I am amazed at how the Designer worked out the sexual development of animals, and man, and some plants. How on earth does an animal know instinctively how to copulate? Sometimes the Designer apparently made a mistake when He made a person with the brain of one sex and the genitals of the other. Then there is the curious duck-billed Platypus, with a large duck's bill, an animal-like body, and the ability to lay eggs and then have the embryo come down (too soon?) and reside there in a pouch until it is ready to be born. There is an odd one!

No one can know who the Designer was. (Or were there a long series of designers?) If there were a series of designers, we do not know where or how they got their astounding mastery of chemistry, where they may have had their laboratory, where they lived, or why they were so devoted to their work.

What I marvel most at is how they could have given such remarkable instincts to living things. How, for instance, does a mother bird or seal in a crowded group of hundreds recognize her child? How does the mother know how to feed and take care of her young? How does a human newborn infant know enough to suck at its mother's nipples? It is remarkable that a little bird called the Plover knows enough to leave the Aleutian Island chain bordering the Bering Sea and make its way to the Hawaiian Islands. I wonder also how many birds and other animals know where and how to find their source of food. How do the carnivores know which animal to hunt,and how to deceive it, and in reverse, how do many animals know how to evade so skillfully the predators wich hunt them?

The most wonderful organ, of course, is the brain — particularly the human brain. It is said to contain approximately a billion cells! I marvel that I can recall many scenes which I saw when I was only three years old. How is it that I can remember, in detail, conversations that I had when I was a boy. I recently heard some music which I remembered well, even though the last time I heard that music was when I was in Hawaii just before going to college in 1901! I sometimes wonder if evolution will continue from this time on. I do not see why it could not. (But if the tendency of ignorant people is to have many children and the tendency of gifted people is to have few cildren or none at all, the future could be bad.) As time passes, perhaps the big apes will learn more sophisticated social behavior, and even be able to talk!

One thing that I am happy and hopeful about is that evolution is still taking place in the sciences and in medicine. Fifty years ago I could easily read a medical or scientific journal from cover to cover, but now medicine and science in general have become so technical that I, who used to be a laboratory researcher, can only read with difficulty many of the journals. Doubtless in time the language of medicine and science will constantly get more technical.

I have been glad to find that thousands of people who do not want more children are now having themselves sterilized. This practice can be very helpful. In a fine book by Dr. Curtis Woods Jr. *Sex Without Babies: A Comprehensive Review of Voluntary Sterilization as a Method of Birth Control,* I found a remarkable photograph of an unpleasant, markedly feeble-minded woman accompanied by the statement that she had had sixteen equally feeble-minded children, who in turn produced thirty-two mentally retarded children. Not one of the forty-eight offspring was able to learn to read! Imagine how much money her city could have saved by having that woman sterilized before she had the 48 offspring who all their days will cost the city thousands of dollars a year. Another odd thing — many years ago while travelling, I saw an unfortunate little woman who, like a hominid, had a small skull with a retreating forehead and a prominent lower jaw that suggested the snout of an ape! She had an ancient type of skull.

One thing about the Designer is that although He has been kind and even idealistic at times, He has also been, it seems, needlessly cruel and murderous. This is true in the case of the useless mosquito, most species of which are bad enough, making sleep almost impossible in some areas of the world. But some species of mosquito have killed thousands of people in Asia, and perhaps over a million people in the world. One of the worst curses of mankind was the Black Death, a form of plague transmitted by infected rats that was pandemic throughout Europe and much of Asia in the years 1347 through 1353. This murderous disease killed off as much as one third of the population of Europe! And until recent years the poliomyelitis germ was so very cruel, because, as we all know, it tended to strike thousands of defenseless children, leaving them paralyzed and unhappy.

I have always felt that there is a wealth of evidence to show that the Designer continued to learn over countless centuries, and He continually improved the living things that He made. Curiously, on most islands of the world, there are few animals, and usually there are no large mammals. When the English arrived in Australia, there were no mammals other than some bats and rats and the remarkable monotremes whose females keep their young for a time in a pouch. It is also curious that in the island of Borneo, there are a few apes. Perhaps long ago a couple were brought there by travelers. Another odd fact is that a few years ago, as most of us know, some religious groups fought to keep their children from being taught about evolution in school.

My feeling is that, because in the last hundred million years there have been so many splendid improvements in animals and men, we can look forward to the coming of many more improvements in the future.

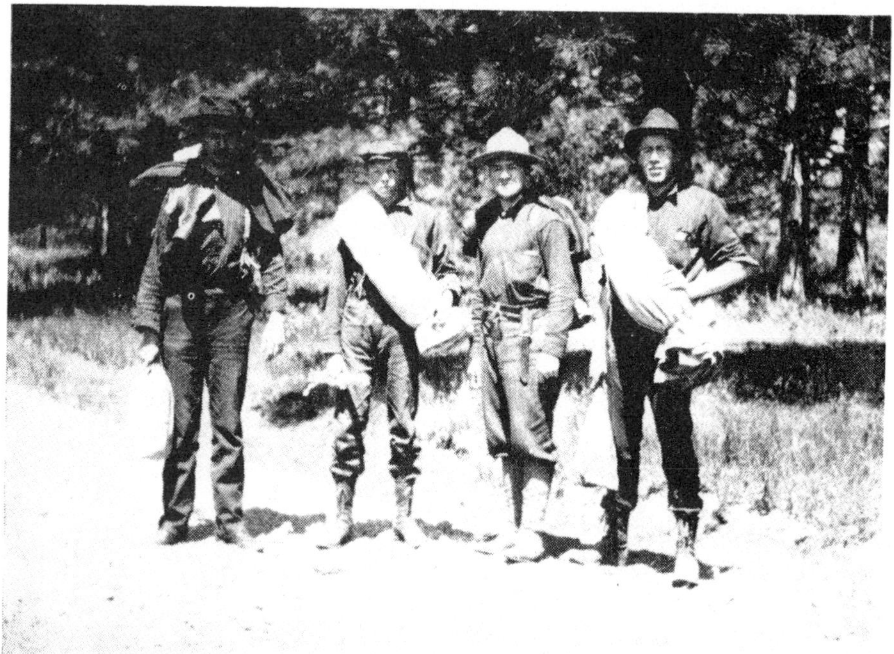

My first Sierra Club trip — May, 1905. "Happy" Reed, William Smyth, "Judd" Harris, and me

POST SCRIPT

I hope this book has given an adequate picture of the career of a physician through three quarters of this most remarkable century. My hope is that it has clearly portrayed my life, my ideals, and the work I have loved to do. It will have done what I hoped if it improves the relations between laymen and physicians, and serve as a stimulus to doctors and idealistic medical students to live a life dedicated to both the art and science of medicine and public health.

And finally, it is my hope that through my text there shines forth my lifelong love and devotion to medicine, as well as my love for others.